ELEGANT ELEVATION

SHATTERING THROUGH THE
GLASS CEILING TO BECOME
THE BEST VERSION OF YOU

Michelle R. Williams

WESTBOW
PRESS®
A DIVISION OF THOMAS NELSON
& ZONDERVAN

WestBow Press books may be ordered through booksellers or by contacting:

WestBow Press
A Division of Thomas Nelson & Zondervan
1663 Liberty Drive
Bloomington, IN 47403
www.westbowpress.com
844-714-3454

Scripture quotations taken from The Holy Bible, New International
Version® NIV® Copyright © 1973 1978 1984 2011 by Biblica,
Inc. TM. Used by permission. All rights reserved worldwide.

ISBN: 978-1-6642-6132-7 (sc)
ISBN: 978-1-6642-6134-1 (hc)
ISBN: 978-1-6642-6133-4 (e)

Library of Congress Control Number: 2022905077

Print information available on the last page.

WestBow Press rev. date: 04/18/2022

CONTENTS

Dedication.. vii
Introduction ix

Chapter 1   Faith 1
Chapter 2   Intermittent Fasting 10
Chapter 3   God's Favor.. 16

Phase I   Stop the Bleeding & Find the Source......................20
Phase II   Remove the Debris and Purify Your Heart.............22

Chapter 4   Generational Curses...24
Chapter 5   Abandonment/Loss...30
Chapter 6   Self-Image/Self Love..38
Chapter 7   Overcoming Trauma 45
Chapter 8   Mental Health Issues 59
Chapter 9   Parental Guilt 70
Chapter 10   Acceptance & the Unconditional Love of God.......73

Phase III   Change & Rebuild Your Core...............................84
Phase IV   Strengthen Your Faith to Become the Best
              Version of You 89

Conclusion 105
Acknowledgements.. 107

DEDICATION

I dedicate this book to my mother. Although in this book I discuss some of the tough love that you displayed to me and challenging times that we shared, I would not have traded you for anything. You were my best friend in the entire world. You gave me three of the best gifts that you could ever give someone; The knowledge of God, life and the best of you. Thank you for all of the stories that you shared and for making me read and write reports from the Encyclopedia Britannica collection when I misbehaved. It truly expanded my knowledge and vocabulary, which both were extremely helpful as I wrote this book. I hope that following my dreams has made you smile and filled your heart with joy. I love you mama and miss you dearly.

INTRODUCTION

Thank you in advance for taking the time to read my book. I pray that it will bless your soul and have a lasting positive impact on your life. I am confident that it will help guide you in your personal journey of shattering through the glass ceiling to become the best version of you. My name is Michelle Williams. I am a Certified Holistic Wellness Coach, Visionary Leader and Author. I have a Bachelor of Science Degree in Business Management and a Project Management Certification, but my true passion is striving to be a significant part of the change that I wish to see in the world. I want to help other people overcome life's obstacles and barriers by introducing the same program that helped me become the best version of myself. The name of the program is Elegant Elevation. The Elegant Elevation program helped me to uncover underlying issues and tackle the root cause instead of focusing on minor symptoms that could be seen on the surface of my life. This book provides a guide on how to incorporate holistic wellness into your life to become the best version of you.

My inspiration and motivation to write this book came from losing both of my parents and many other loved ones prematurely to preventable health conditions such as congestive heart failure and diabetes. Over the years, I discovered that many of my loved ones met this tragic fate due to lack of knowledge about the factors that contributed to and caused high blood pressure, congestive heart failure and diabetes such as inadequate sleep, consuming significantly more food than their body needed to function (and consuming it too often), living a sedentary lifestyle, not properly managing the stress in their lives and failing to adopt a holistic approach to wellness.

I developed the Elegant Elevation program because I wholeheartedly believe in achieving overall wellness through a holistic approach which includes the Mind, Body and Spirit. We need for each one of these "buckets" to be full in our lives in order to be healthy. I struggled with my weight for most of my adult life. I could always manage to lose weight but could never sustain the weight loss. The reason I could never sustain my weight loss is because I was approaching my issue with weight as if it were the actual problem. When truthfully the excess weight was just a symptom of several underlying issues that I needed to resolve. It wasn't until I was able to identify and uncover those underlying issues that caused me to overeat and gain weight in the first place, that I was able to live and maintain a healthier lifestyle and weight. I am dedicated and committed to helping you do the same.

Let me begin with why I named the program, book and brand Elegant Elevation. Some of the words and synonyms in the dictionary used to describe "Elegant" are refined, classy, graceful, distinguished, charming, dignified and exquisite. Often when we are going through a phase of transformation, we view the result that we want to achieve as the destination or "grand prize." But we fail to acknowledge, appreciate, and celebrate the process, journey, and season that we are currently in and persevering through. We are refined, classy, graceful, distinguished, charming, dignified and exquisite just as we are. Right here and right now, we are all of the words that define and describe "elegant." It doesn't matter if we are male or female, Black or White, young, or old. We are "elegant." We do not have to wait until we reach our goal of becoming the best version of ourselves to acknowledge, appreciate and celebrate ourselves, our qualities, our gifts, and our elegance.

We live in a time where instant gratification and overnight success is the goal and is celebrated. We often skip right over that middle part; the process that it took for us to attain success. If the process is in fact mentioned, we often refer to it as the struggle or hard times instead of the beautiful growing or awakening transformation that it is. We often tend to glaze right over that part of the story. That part is where we gained the most knowledge through trial and error. It is where we increased our faith because that is all we had to carry us through. It is often the part where we strengthened our relationship with God because we could not trust our own instincts and judgment. We had to rely solely on His guidance. That is the part of the story that we need to share more than either the starting point or the ending when we reach our goals or achieve our dreams. We need to share every one of those lessons that we learned. We need to share how God made a way out of no way. That is the most useful part of the journey that others need to hear above all. That is the part of our story that others can apply to their own lives to achieve their goals and dreams, since their starting point or beginning may drastically differ from ours. They may not be able to see how our story and journey is similar to theirs because the other circumstances in their lives are so different.

The definition of elevation is the action or fact of elevating or being elevated to a higher level, which is exactly what happens when you apply faith, intermittent fasting and God's favor to your life to achieve holistic wellness and become the best version of you. I included "Shattering through the Glass Ceiling" in the title of the book to illustrate the barriers and obstacles that we all encounter that force us to rely on our faith and God's favor to shatter through and overcome. Each one of us has our own set of barriers and obstacles that we need to shatter through and overcome to get to the other side to become the best version of ourselves.

In this book, I will share with you some of the most painful barriers and challenging obstacles that I had to shatter through and overcome to become the best version of myself. This process is not a destination, but a journey. Elegant Elevation is a program that encompasses Faith, Intermittent Fasting and God's Favor. It helps you learn how to use God's word, His grace and His mercy to overcome the obstacles and barriers that are preventing you from becoming the best version of you. As I continue my walk with God and on my personal voyage, I will continue to assess my circumstances, evaluate myself and apply the principles I have learned and used to develop Elegant Elevation to ensure that I am constantly growing and evolving. I hope after reading this book that you will do the same in your life.

CHAPTER
1

FAITH

MY UNDERSTANDING AND DEFINITION OF FAITH IS A FIRM BELIEF, strong conviction, complete trust and reliance on God. Prior to writing this book, I had to develop my faith that God would lead me through each step of this process. I had to increase my faith in my ability to trust, honor and obey Him completely. I had to have faith that although I decided to publish my book through a Christian publishing company that this message could and would reach people from all denominations and walks of life. I had to have absolute faith in God to ensure that I did not let my personal fears stand in the way of a message that needed to be shared. As you read this book and begin to apply its principles, you will need to have faith that you can reach your goals to become the best version of you. Your goal may be weight-loss, improved self-care or to start fully operating in your gift. Despite what your goals may be, it is imperative that you have complete faith that God can and will help you achieve them.

When I told my husband and some of my close family members about the personal content I planned to share in this book they asked me if I was worried about being so transparent. They asked if I had considered how others may look at me differently and judge me after they read my book. I responded quickly and honestly that I was not worried. God did not create me worry. He created me to do His will and fulfill His purpose for my life. I wholeheartedly believe that my purpose is to help others by sharing my journey. I have always believed that we exhaust too much energy worrying about what others will think of us instead of following our hearts and having faith in God and his will for our lives.

I look at everyone in the world as puzzle pieces to a beautiful, enormous and complete picture. Alone we are imperfect and incomplete, but if we put our puzzle pieces and gifts together, we can be a whole and perfect picture. God gave us all precious gifts or essential puzzle pieces that we can and should use to help others to complete the picture. Sometimes, instead of us appreciating one another's gifts and sharing our own, we look down on these gifts and pass judgment, possibly believing that the gifts that we possess cause us to be superior or inferior. We may believe that the gifts that God blessed us with are more or less valuable than the gifts he has blessed others with.

This is so untrue and is not God's will for us. God blessed me with the gifts of compassion, empathy and writing. He also gave me an assignment to share the lessons that I have learned on my journey with others. I will do everything in my power to fulfill it, even if I am judged or looked down upon because of it. If my journey helps someone else elevate and have a better quality of life, then it was worth it. I cannot allow myself to be concerned with what other people may think, feel or say about me for sharing my journey. I also will not let it prevent me from completing the assignment that He gave me to fulfill. I had to have faith that if God brought me to it, He would bring me through it.

I can clearly recall an assistant pastor at my former church preaching a sermon one Sunday on repentance. He mentioned in that sermon that we should stop judging and condemning each other, especially when a person has repented for their wrongdoing. He said that for everyone in the sanctuary that day there was someone who could walk through the church doors at that very moment and make them drop their heads in shame because they know something about them that they were ashamed of and did not want anyone else to ever know. That statement always remained in the back of my mind and reminded me to remain humble and not judge others because it was a true and accurate statement. (Keeping this statement in mind helped give me the courage to share some of the intimate details in this book.)

When I began coaching and people began to share their pain, struggles and regrets with me, I realized just how accurate that statement was. So if others choose to judge me because I am human, imperfect, made some mistakes and bad decisions, then I have no choice but to allow them to do so. That just means this book is not intended for them. This book is for people who embrace the fact that they are imperfect beings who may have some issues that need to be resolved and have the desire to grow and develop into the best version of themselves. They realize that they can learn from the knowledge, experience and journeys of others. I am writing this book for those individuals who will take the information and resources they need from this book and apply them to their own lives to elevate themselves to the best version possible.

I decided to write this book in this format because I believe there is a need for this type of content, and information and I wanted to fulfill that need. My former pastor, spiritual leader and someone who I proudly call a friend often spoke about how Christians and God's people in general needed to have a servant's heart. He encouraged the members of the church to get involved in a ministry. He stated that every one of us had been given a gift and should use that gift to serve others and God in some capacity. He went on to say that even if we did not feel that our gift could be used in any of the existing ministries at the church, we could start a new ministry by simply finding a need and fulfilling it. I believe that God put the desire and need to share my journey in my heart and I had to have faith that He will give me all of the tools that I need to achieve that.

In addition to having faith in God. I also had to have faith in myself. I had to believe that God had blessed me with everything that I needed to write this book, share my journey and help others to elevate to the best versions of themselves. When I began my weight loss journey over 20 years ago, I read every article about weight loss in every magazine and every book that I could find on the subject. I watched every infomercial, documentary, video and movie that I came across on the topic of weight loss and obesity. I attended workshops and conferences on weight loss. I tried different supplements and medications that claimed to burn body fat and help to suppress hunger and food cravings. Due to my determination to be healthy and lose weight, I was always committed to each diet or plan that I tried. As a result of my determination, I always had some level of success and would lose what some would consider a significant amount of weight within a reasonably short period of time.

I would always couple exercise with whatever plan I was following. So, I would often walk on my breaks and lunch periods while at work. I would also walk and complete a workout after coming home from work. Family, friends, and some members from my church would ask what I was doing to lose weight. I was always eager to share whatever plan I was on and the exercise regime I was following. I wanted to inspire as many others as I could to become healthy as well, so I created and led several health and weight loss challenges at work to encourage my coworkers to embrace healthy eating and exercise.

I also participate in several annual community fundraiser events such as the Susan G. Komen Race for the Cure and the American Heart Association Heart Walk, which are events that raise awareness and funds for research to fight and cure breast cancer and heart disease. I always volunteer to be a team captain and try to encourage as many people as I can to sign up and participate because this is a great way to help others, be a part of the solution and be active at the same time. In addition to trying to follow a healthy eating plan and exercising, I always tried to ensure that I sought out positive and uplifting content to read, watch and listen to. I would watch and listen to tons of diverse inspirational, encouraging, motivational, and spiritual programs, YouTube videos, and podcasts. I would read similar types of books.

I learned an abundance of information from these sources. There are too many to name, but some of my absolute favorite people to watch, read and listen to in no particular order are Joyce Meyer, Bishop TD Jakes, Sarah Jakes Roberts, Joel Osteen, Les Brown, Devon Franklin, Oprah Winfrey, Steve Harvey, Mel Robbins, Tabitha Brown and Trent Shelton.

In addition to these sources, I would also watch comedy and listen to a wide variety of music. I know this may be frowned upon by some believers because they may believe that Christians should not listen to or watch anything "secular" but I genuinely believe that laughter is good for the soul and God can speak to you through various sources if your heart, outlook and motives are pure. Although some of the comedy that I listen to occasionally has some "questionable" content or profanity, I am able to filter that out and listen for the positive message or lessons that can be found in this type of material. I truly believe Mark 7:15 confirms this way of thinking: "Nothing outside a person can defile them by going into them. Rather it is what comes out of a person that defiles them." I understand that this scripture was referencing the sacred ceremonial practice of washing hands prior to consuming food. It illustrates that anything that enters our bodies through our mouths, passes through our stomachs, doesn't penetrate our heart, is eliminated from our bodies and does not defile us. But I believe the wisdom in this scripture can be used and applied to a plethora of scenarios including the secular content we sometimes see or hear. If we are looking through a spiritual lens and allowing the Holy Spirit to work in us, these things will not penetrate our hearts or defile us.

Listening and watching some secular content has helped me to stay in touch with what is going on in the world. If I am going to fulfill my purpose, be about God's work, and fulfill a need, I believe I need to know what is going on in the world to identify what those specific needs are. A perfect example of hearing a spiritual word in secular content is one day I was traveling to be with a dear friend who was having major surgery for a serious health condition. I was a nervous wreck due to the circumstances surrounding why I was making the drive. In addition, I get uneasy about driving on the highway due to the number of people who are distracted and drive recklessly at times.

The fact that my friend who was going through this terrible ordeal is only a few years older than me did not help matters. She and I have a close relationship. She is such a strong and funny woman. We are both just big kids at heart, especially when we get together. When we visit each other (we reside in different states) she and I often listen or watch comedy online or on TV. We take turns sharing videos, shows or movies of our favorite comedians.

I had just lost my mother a couple of years prior so I was secretly afraid of losing another loved one. I prayed and listened to some music and YouTube videos with spiritual content. Listening to the music and videos with spiritual content slightly improved my mood, but I was still feeling down. I continued to drive, trying not to become petrified by the way cars were speeding and swerving around me.

I was doing the exact speed limit of 65 MPH and refused to go a mile faster. I was reminiscing about the fun times she and I had shared together. It was like I could literally see and hear her laugh. She always gave great advice. I wondered what advice she might have given me if this situation involved another close friend or family member. I instantly knew that she would tell me that I need to listen to something that would lighten my mood and make me laugh.

I was listening to gospel music on Pandora radio and I quickly switched to a comedy station. I would say that I was shocked at what I heard coming through the speakers of my car, but I know that God operates in ways that can appear extremely mysterious to us, so I wasn't shocked one bit. I just smiled to myself and praised God for being who He is, when I realized that a comedian by the name of Eddie Griffin was in the middle of doing a set on Christians, Muslims, the Bible, Jesus, and religion. For those who may believe that it is a sin to listen to anything with secular content, I apologize in advance for my next statement, but the set was hilarious. My mood drastically improved by just listening to the comedic set. I instantly felt significantly more relaxed. I thought about how much my friend would have enjoyed listening to this comedian.

Eddie was discussing how Muslims and Christians debate about who the "messenger" was. He stated that Christians believe that Jesus was the "messenger" and he said that Muslims believe that Mohammad was the "messenger." He went on to say, "I say who cares who the messenger is, did you get the message?" He shared that he didn't understand why we battle so much about religion when the general consensus is the same, do unto others as you will have them do to you and to have the knowledge and discernment to be able to decipher right from wrong.

Although, I am a Christian I have friends who are Catholic, Jehovah's Witness, Muslim, and Seventh-Day Adventist. I have often witnessed these debates over religion and beliefs and also wondered why we spent so much time trying to convince each other that our religion was the right one instead of appreciating each other's different beliefs and just focusing on doing God's will and His work. I have so many more things in common with these friends than differences and was not going to allow our different religious beliefs prevent us from being friends. We all believed in God and were all people who wanted to fulfill God's purpose for us.

It was at that moment that I completely understood why our pastor used to always say "One God, One Faith." My pastor had said that very statement hundreds if not thousands of times at service on Sunday morning. I heard him each time that he said it but it took the way that the comedian delivered that message for me to truly grasp the entirety and meaning of what message my pastor was trying to convey by saying those words.

Yes, the comedian did use some profanity and made light of some of the Bible scriptures, but I did not retain any of that. I knew that he was a believer in God, and he was using his gift of having the ability to make people laugh to relay a positive and important message. What I retained from that comedic skit that had a positive impact on my life and how I viewed other people and their religious beliefs was that it does not matter if someone has a different religion or belief than I do. We can still work together to fulfill God's purpose and plan for our lives and the world, in addition to collaborating to help others fulfill their purpose in the process. I pray that people from all religions will benefit from the information shared in this book. Despite our spiritual and religious beliefs most of us have a genuine desire to be the best versions of ourselves.

Many other "secular"comedians, instructors, coaches, authors, actors and motivational speakers have shared positive messages that have impacted my life. Each of those people have shared information that has helped me to overcome obstacles and broaden my vision and outlook as a woman and a Christian in a different and unique capacity. As I have said and will continue to reiterate throughout this book, God has given everyone, regardless of age, race, gender, religion, sexual orientation, background, or political beliefs a special gift to use to fulfill His will and purpose and to help others. I believe that once we truly embrace and understand that fact, the world will become a much better place.

Faith, intentional positive mental health, and spirituality were always large components in my life. What I did not realize until much later on in my journey was how closely these components were related to my physical wellness. I learned the importance and need to approach wellness as a holistic effort including mind, body and spirit. I want to help other individuals learn to approach wellness as a holistic effort by using and applying the knowledge that I have gathered over the years through traditional and self-study methods. I have faith and confidence that my education, knowledge and experience well equipped me to do this.

I have mentioned the need to have faith in God and ourselves, but we must also have faith in the process that it takes to achieve our goals and become the best versions of ourselves. Having faith in the process is just as significant in achieving our goals as having faith in God and ourselves. Regardless of whether we believe that the process will work or it will not work, we are right. We can only achieve what we believe. If we have doubts that a process will work, it usually won't because we do not have faith that it will and we are not giving our full effort. When I began intermittent fasting to lose weight, I had faith that it would work to help me lose those extra pounds for good and it did!

CHAPTER
2

❀

INTERMITTENT FASTING

I MENTIONED EARLIER THAT I STRUGGLED WITH MY WEIGHT FOR MANY years. I tried just about every diet known to man including Atkins, Slim Fast, Weight Watchers, Lean Cuisine, Jenny Craig, low fat, counting calories, smoothie diets and cleanses just to name a few. I found minimal success with each one of these diets. They all worked until they didn't. I believe that every diet can work for someone but no one diet works for everyone. I would often lose 20, 30, or even 40 pounds, then become exhausted with the diet and start to feel deprived. I would revert to previous eating habits and the weight would eventually pile back on. I would gain back the weight that I lost and usually a few (or more than a few) extra pounds. I would feel discouraged and defeated and start the cycle all over again and begin the search for the next miracle diet.

After spending 20+ years yo-yo dieting, I discovered Intermittent Fasting which helped me to lose weight yet again. However, the weight was just a symptom of some much larger underlying issues. If I did not address those issues, the weight loss like many times before, would be short lived. During my many years of yo-yo dieting, I often kept a log of my food intake and exercise. Prior to discovering Intermittent Fasting, I still had the mindset that managing the calories in versus calories out was the recipe to lose weight. I believed if I burned more calories than I consumed than I would automatically lose weight. I was so wrong and we will discuss the errors in that theory throughout this book. In the latter years of my yo-yo dieting, in addition to keeping a record of my food intake and exercise habits, I began to keep a journal.

In the beginning, I started journaling primarily to keep a record of my weight loss progress, what foods I was eating and how my body responded to those foods. I later purchased a Fitbit fitness tracker that kept track of my exercise, heart rate, steps per day, weight, macronutrients, (carbohydrates, fats and protein) water intake and sleep habits. I loved having all this valuable data at my fingertips. I also began to log all of this information in my journal. When I began to Intermittent Fast, I jumped head first into the lifestyle by choosing the eating style of one meal a day or (OMAD). Intermittent Fasting offers many different fasting style options and windows. But I fell into the one meal a day eating style naturally because I was not hungry in the morning and when I ate lunch in the middle of the day, I would become extremely sleepy around 2 or 3 PM. I would then struggle to focus for the remainder of the workday or be productive for the remainder of the day on weekends.

I will usually fast for 20-22 hours each day and consume all my food for the day within a two to four hour eating window. During my two to four hour eating window, I do not follow any strict diets or eating plans. I also do not count calories anymore or eliminate entire food groups. However, I try to make healthier food choices. My diet primarily consists of fish, chicken, vegetables, fruit, complex carbohydrates, and plenty of unsweetened green tea, black coffee and H2O.

Although I did not eliminate any complete food groups, I did drastically limit my intake of overly processed foods (anything frozen, or in a box or can), junk food such as chips, candy, cookies, and fast food. While I did no longer count calories, I made sure not to overeat, overindulge or consume more calories than my body needed. That is where the fruit of the spirit self-control comes into play and must be implemented. While I could easily eat an entire family bag of chips or an entire row of cookies, my body did not need all of that and I understood that it was not a healthy choice to excessively consume all of that processed food and sugar. I could be just as satisfied with having a handful of chips or a couple of cookies on occasion.

This eating plan worked well for me. I was able to lose over 70 pounds in about six months. I know that most of the weight that I lost initially was due to inflammation, bloating, water weight and being insulin resistant but it still felt great to be relieved of the excess pounds. Intermittent Fasting gives your body a break from constantly consuming and digesting food. It gives your body the opportunity to tap into your body's fat stores for energy instead of using the foods that we consume throughout the day for fuel.

I noticed as I was logging my food that some days I seemed to be much hungrier than others and would consume more food. I also noticed that there were days that I seemed to crave specifically more sweets and processed foods than usual. This finding piqued my interest and prompted me to try to find out why this was happening. Once I discover that something is happening, I need to find out the reason why. I have discovered that if I can find out why something happens, I can usually find a resolution to the problem or issue.

Discovering that there were certain days that I felt hungrier or desired more "junk food" than usual, prompted me to start adding how I was feeling and my mental state in my daily journal entry. I had heard many times over the years during my study of weight loss and obesity that our mood and mental state can have an impact on what type or how much food we crave and consume. I was also familiar with the term "emotional eating." After a few weeks of logging my daily emotional and mental state, I identified a couple of patterns.

The first pattern I noticed was the weather had a huge impact on my mood, mental state and eating habits. On days when it was cold, rainy and/or gloomy, I felt lethargic and lacked motivation. I did not engage in as much exercise or other activities and I also craved and ate more "junk food" than usual. On days that I experienced more work related or personal stress, I also ate more and engaged in less exercise and activities. On the days when the weather was not as favorable or that I experienced more stress, my sleep schedule was also impacted, which sometimes caused me to overeat or crave more "junk food" the following day. In addition, on the days of my monthly menstrual cycle, I also consumed more food and craved more "junk food."

Now that I had discovered why I ate more on certain days than others, I needed to devise a plan to choose an alternative option other than food to cope with my emotions and stress levels. Since I did not have any control over the weather, the power to completely eliminate stress, emotions or my monthly menstrual cycle, I had to find other ways to combat and deal with these situations in a more productive manner. I was reverting to food, not because I was hungry, but because I was using food to resolve an issue that I should have used my faith and God's word to aid me in overcoming. Instead of using food to cope when I begin to feel overwhelmed, stressed, or depressed, I now meditate on God's word or seek inspiration to overcome these stressors.

Overeating is not a healthy coping mechanism and causes me to gain excess weight which can lead to more serious health issues and eventually even death as it did with my parents and many other loved ones. Overeating and obesity can and often will lead to heart disease, diabetes or stroke. Intermittent Fasting offers many health benefits as it relates to obesity, heart health and diabetes. Since beginning an Intermittent Lifestyle my LDL ("bad cholesterol"), blood pressure and glucose levels have all drastically been reduced. But I still have to do my part to manage my eating habits even when my window is open to ensure that I do not consume more calories daily than my body needs. One of my favorite scriptures to meditate on is James 1:2-4. "Consider it pure joy, my brothers and sisters, whenever you face trials of many kinds, because you know that the testing of your faith produces perseverance. Let perseverance finish its work so that you may be mature and complete, not lacking anything."

I love this scripture because it changed my perspective of what I was going through. Instead of feeling sorry for myself and feeling deprived because I recognized that I could no longer overindulge in unhealthy foods, this scripture verifies that this is not true. It tells me that I am getting stronger in these times. Times such as these allow me to trust in God and His Word and understand if I can persevere through these situations, I am growing and maturing in my Christian walk. I am not an infant or child, I do not have to overindulge in food or other unhealthy activities to try to achieve instant gratification or relief from my situation. I can have peace, be still in my situation and have confidence through my faith that our God is working it out behind the scenes and I am growing in the process. I want to be whole, complete and lacking nothing as indicated in His word. Learning to have self-control with food consumption is a minor inconvenience and growing pain that is necessary in achieving that next level of maturity in my journey. It may not be easy all the time, but it is definitely worth it to become the best version of me possible.

We all have different obstacles and barriers that we will have to overcome to become the best versions of ourselves. However, the answer to shattering through these barriers will be the same. The answer can be found through having faith in our God and His word. God and His word are the same today, tomorrow and forevermore. Psalm 37:5 truly helped me to get out of my own way and go to God and His word for answers to any problem or issue that I face. "Commit your way to the Lord; trust in Him and He will do this."

It is so important that we get and stay out of our own way. God has the answers to life's problems and issues. He has shared and given us access to these answers through His word. He has also given us the power of discernment through the Holy Spirit. We truly need to rely more on God, His Word, and the Holy Spirit to address the barriers and obstacles that we face daily. We make it so much harder on ourselves, by trying to take matters into our own hands. And honestly, we usually end up compounding the issue and making the situation even worse.

Rarely are we resorting to overeating or engaging in other unhealthy vices such as gambling, smoking, drinking, substance use, promiscuity, pornography, gossiping and judging due to a necessity or just because we enjoy engaging in these activities that much. We often use food and the other vices mentioned above to do one of three things: We use these vices to either soothe a wound, fill a void/satisfy a feeling of emptiness or to escape our current situation. Each one of these issues can be resolved by having faith in God and His Word. I have found that Intermittent Fasting is a great tool to prevent using food and eating as an escape to avoid dealing with stress and other issues.

CHAPTER
3

❧

GOD'S FAVOR

Many of us have had to endure and try to overcome obstacles in life such as extreme loss, mental health issues, trauma, abuse, generational curses, poverty and intellectual or physical disabilities. I had to shatter through some of these barriers to become the best version of me. I have not always chosen the healthiest options to try to cope with these issues. If we are honest, most of us have indulged in at least one or more unhealthy vices to attempt to bury the issues that often haunt us and disrupt our peace of mind. Prior to developing a true relationship with God and increasing my faith in His word, I selected various unhealthy options to cope with my emotions and feelings. The good news is that when I finally did establish a true and personal relationship with God and started to seek his Word and guidance on how to deal with my issues, I was able to shatter through each one of these barriers and overcome every obstacle that came my way.

I had to pray to God to help me learn how to deny my fleshly desires to resort to these vices, listen to the Holy Spirit and apply God's word in these situations. I find great strength and guidance in reading Galatians 5:16-17- "So I say walk by the Spirit, and you will not gratify these desires of the flesh. For the flesh desires what is contrary to the Spirit and the Spirit what is contrary to the flesh. They are in conflict with each other, so that you are not able to do whatever you want."

I always feel convicted, when I operate from flesh instead of the Holy Spirit. I have learned to take a pause before I act to allow the Holy Spirit to lead me and direct my steps. When I faced a barrier or obstacle, I started to include God in the equation by praying about the situation and then seeking out a scripture in the Bible that addressed the situation that I was dealing with. Usually after I pray about the situation, (sometimes I must deny the desire to become overly anxious and ensure that I am exercising patience) God will place the answer in my heart or direct my attention to a scripture in the Bible. Sometimes I will be proactive and start reading the Bible directly after I pray. This always soothes me, and I am usually led to the answer to the issue I am dealing with. Having the ability to deny my flesh and allow my faith in God and the Holy Spirit to lead me did not happen overnight. It definitely is a process and takes some effort and discipline. I am human so denying my flesh is still a daily battle.

God's favor is an essential part of how I overcame obstacles and barriers to become the best version of me. I understand favor to be one way God demonstrates his love for us by blessing us and giving us preferential treatment as his children in certain situations. I believe that each of the steps that I took also helped to increase God's favor in my life. I believe in order to increase God's favor we must at a minimum follow these three steps: (1) Listen to God and the Holy Spirit, (2) Trust Him/Have Faith in His Power (3) Obey His Word. The more that I followed these steps, the more that I witnessed His favor in my life. I began to receive blessings and opportunities that I knew could only be His favor. In addition to praying and being obedient to His word, having God's favor can help us navigate those challenging obstacles and barriers that we face in life to become the best version of ourselves.

There are four phases in the process that I completed in conjunction with faith, Intermittent Fasting and God's favor to help me learn to reject my flesh and become the best version of me.

It was interesting how God revealed each step that I needed to take in this process. This was just another example of the Holy Spirit and His favor working in my life. It is nothing less than amazing from where or from whom we may receive a message or an answer from God about the issues we are praying about. In addition, it is also extremely important that we have an open mind and heart to things and people that we encounter. You never know, God may provide your answer through something or someone that you would normally disregard. I often think of Hebrews 13:2. "Do not forget to show hospitality to strangers, for by doing so some people have shown hospitality to angels without knowing it."

One day, when I had just finished my morning prayer and reading my daily word on the Our Daily Bread app on my phone I saw the title "Wound Care" in my phone's search history. I thought to myself this is odd. I don't recall why I would have been searching for wound care on the internet. Although I have several family members who work in the healthcare industry, I could not imagine why they may have been searching for wound care on the internet while at my home visiting and connected to the Wi-Fi. Despite not initially knowing how or why this title had appeared in my search bar, I felt the inclination to click on the title and review the first item that came up in the results. It was titled How Wounds Heal: The 4 Main Phases to Wound Healing.

Before having a personal relationship with God, I may have said, "For some reason I felt compelled to continue to read through this document." But now that I have a personal relationship with Him, I know that he can send messages through many different sources. I know that He has usually spoken to me through something I am reading, watching, or listening to. I know that the reason that I was compelled to continue to read through this document was because there was a message or an answer from Him somewhere in the contents. Before I continue, I want to back up for just a second and share that my morning prayer had included a plea for God to remove the things from me that are not like Him or of His will. I also prayed that he creates in me a clear mind and clean heart. I prayed for Him to heal me in the places that I was broken and that he would clearly reveal to me His purpose for my life and the steps that I needed to take to be in alignment with His plan and begin to move in that direction. I did not know if I was being led to read this document to uncover a message or answer for that prayer, or a completely different issue. It really didn't matter, because I was sure that either way there was something significant that I was going to find, so I continued to read through the document.

This document listed that the four main phases to healing a wound in bold letters were: Phase I-Hemostasis Phase, Phase II: Defensive/Inflammatory Phase, Phase III: Proliferative Phase and Phase IV: Maturation Phase. At first glance, although I had seen most of these words before, I did not know exactly what each phase meant and entailed so I continued to read through the document and discovered that the Hemostasis Phase meant to "stop the bleeding." The Defensive/Inflammatory Phase meant to focus on "destroying the bacteria." The Proliferative Phase means to "fill and cover the wound." The Maturation Phase means the new tissue has grown over the wound and this new tissue is slowly "gaining strength and flexibility." God revealed to me that these phases were very similar to the steps that I would need to take in order to heal from my past. (These underlying wounds and issues were the reason that I over ate and would always regain the weight after I lost it.) I would need to complete each one of these phases to shatter through the barriers, overcome the obstacles that had been holding me back, to stop self-sabotaging and allowing my flesh to lead me astray and to begin to fully operate in the spirit of God to become the best version of me. The following scripture gave me the confidence and strength to do just that (Psalm 147:3 "He heals the brokenhearted and binds up their wounds").

PHASE

I

STOP THE BLEEDING
& FIND THE SOURCE

EACH PHASE OF THIS PROCESS TO BECOME THE BEST VERSION OF ME WAS challenging but vital. The stop the bleeding phase included multiple steps. I needed to start by identifying the source of my pain and completely give that pain over to my source of power and healing, who is none other than God. I had to determine if the situation that caused the pain was a self-inflicted wound or a wound caused by something or someone else. It was essential to know this because I either had to forgive myself or forgive someone else and remember the situation no more. Of course, naturally I will still remember what happened because I am human, but for my spiritual well-being I can no longer ponder over it constantly and allow it to be a barrier or obstacle in my life.

I had many things that were the source of my pain or discomfort throughout my life that I continued to ponder about and allowed to be a barrier or obstacle that delayed my progress in my journey to becoming the best version of me. I created a list of these barriers and obstacles. This was my ceremonial way of shifting my energy and removing these unpleasant memories, thoughts and feelings from my heart, mind, and spirit. I recalled at least 100 different situations that caused me pain and discomfort throughout my life. But some of these situations I grouped together and placed in the same category.

After thinking through each situation that had plagued my mind and heart for many years, I came up with several main areas. The categories or areas of my life that I struggled with the most were Generational Curses, Abandonment/Loss, Self-Image/Self-Love, Trauma, Mental Health Issues, Parental Guilt, and Acceptance. Now that I had compiled my list of areas that I with God's help needed to forgive, be forgiven for, or healed from, I had to have the faith that God could and would guide me through this process. I needed to forgive others, forgive myself and thoroughly heal to become the best version of me; the version of me that God intended for me to be. I can now stop the bleeding from these wounds because I have identified the source and will trust that God will provide the necessary healing and forgiveness for my sins as He says in His word. Romans 3:23-25 helped tremendously with Phase I. "For all have sinned and fall short of the glory of God, and all are justified freely by his grace through the redemption that came by Christ Jesus. God presented Christ as a sacrifice of atonement through the shedding of his blood, to be received by faith. He did this to demonstrate his righteousness, because in his forbearance he had left the sins committed beforehand unpunished."

REMOVE THE DEBRIS AND PURIFY YOUR HEART

IN ADDITION TO IDENTIFYING THE AREAS THAT WERE A SOURCE OF MY pain, creating a list of these areas, and asking for God's help to heal me in those areas, I needed to "confess" and acknowledge those areas in an effort to shatter through the barriers and overcome the obstacles. I needed to clear out the debris and remove any of the lingering feelings that those situations left behind. Again, similar to Phase I writing this step out is ceremonial, but critical in moving past the pain and removing the negative energy associated with these situations.

I know that God was working with me spiritually to heal those wounds, but I had to also follow what His word says. I needed to work and operate in alignment with Him (faith without works is dead) to move past my pain, have the confidence to confess my truth and experiences in order to change my mindset about those experiences as illustrated in James 2:22 "You see that his faith and his actions were working together and his faith was made complete by what he did." The power of confessing and acknowledging our sins is also mentioned in I John 1:9 "If we confess our sins, He is faithful and just and will forgive us our sins and purify us from all unrighteousness." Even though some of the issues that I struggled with were beyond my control, I have not always handled them or responded to them in the way that we were instructed to in Luke 6:37 "Do not judge, and you will not be judged. Do not condemn, and you will not be condemned. Forgive, and you will be forgiven." I definitely did not always adhere to His word when it came to not judging or condemning some things and people, especially myself and those who have hurt me over the years.

I had to let His word resonate in my spirit. How could I expect or even ask God, who is a perfect being for His forgiveness for some of the things I have done in my life and have the audacity to feel that I was in a position to not forgive someone for hurting or wronging me. This is because I had added my own value system to sin and wrongdoing. I was an expert at rationalizing the bad choices I made and things that I did. I always had a reason why I had done those things. This was my way of trying to justify my actions. However, in God's eyes sin is sin and the things that I had done were just as bad as the things that had been done to me. Just like I believed I was justified for doing the things that I had done that were not in alignment with God and His word, I am sure that others thought that they had a good reason or justification for what they did as well.

I had to forgive others for what they had done to me, no matter how heinous I felt the action was. It was not mandatory for me to forgive them for their benefit, but forgiving them was necessary in order for me to be able to have a clean and clear heart when I pray to God and ask for his forgiveness for my shortcomings as stated in Mark 11:25 "And when you stand praying, if you hold anything against anyone, forgive them, so that your Father in heaven may forgive you your sins. "The next step in Phase II: Cleaning out the Debris and Purifying My Heart is to confess my truth and the things that I am harboring in my heart that are preventing me from shattering through the glass ceiling to become the best version of me.

CHAPTER
4

❁

GENERATIONAL CURSES

ONE OF THE AREAS THAT I HAVE STRUGGLED WITH THROUGHOUT MY life is what I refer to as generational curses or generational issues. A generational curse can be defined as the cumulative effect on a person of things that their ancestors did, believed or practiced in the past, and a consequence of an ancestor's actions, beliefs, and sins being passed down. I believe that some of the challenges that I faced were passed down through several generations. Issues with poverty, mental health and single parent homes were things that I saw throughout generations. Although I never had the opportunity to meet my great-grandparents or paternal grandparents I was told that they had jobs but struggled financially.

My maternal grandmother had various gifts and talents such as cooking, writing, sewing and drawing but I never knew of her to have a full-time career in the traditional sense. She never learned to drive, owned a vehicle or a home. In her latter years, she moved from her hometown to the city where some of our family members resided. She lived with my aunt until she was in her 70's, became ill, was diagnosed with a serious mental health condition and had to be moved into a nursing care facility to obtain around the clock supervision and care. She remained there until she passed away at the age of 74.

Many of my other family members lived what some would consider meager lifestyles. Some of the younger generation were college educated, had careers and made a decent living. But none of us had a career such as a lawyer or doctor or would be considered "wealthy." We were primarily working or middle class. Our generation worked hard to break the generational curse of poverty in our family.

I believe that due to my humble beginnings that I tried to enter the workforce as quickly as possible to try to earn money in an effort to improve my living conditions and quality of life. However, even after obtaining my degree, certifications, and securing a career, I felt like I was still living paycheck to paycheck. I believe because I did not have much guidance and direction as it relates to selecting a career, entrepreneurship, or general money management, I was just "winging it" and trying to find my way. I had to apply for grants and student loans to attend school, so I started off my adult life with student loan debt and significantly behind the curve on the road to success. My parents did not own their own business or were they a member of any sororities or fraternities so I was unable to take advantage of any of the referral or employment perks and benefits that are often associated with being a part of that circle.

Growing up in poverty throughout my childhood and teenage years made me feel less than and inadequate in the world. I definitely did not receive the blueprint to success or have anything handed down to me. Everything that I learned about money or handling finances I had to learn on my own through trial and error. However, I do truly appreciate my mother stressing the importance of education to me. Despite being intellectually challenged and in classes for students who had learning disabilities throughout her primary and high school years, she graduated and received a high school diploma. She also ensured that I focused on my education and excelled in school.

I can vividly remember her having a set of Encyclopedia

Britannica books. When I would get into trouble, she would make me read a section of one of the volumes of those books and write a report on it. (I did not know how helpful some of the information that I read in those books would be later in life). I was often asked to participate in clubs, programs, and academic competitions in school such as Scholar's Cup. I made a couple of friends by participating in those groups. But, participating in these types of groups also caused me to realize just how impoverished I was when I saw their clothes, homes, or cars that their parents drove to pick them up. This usually led to me feeling down and decreased my already low self-esteem.

I was often teased and bullied in school because I was poor and wore hand-me downs, generic shoes and received free lunch. At the schools that I attended, they called the names of the kids who received free lunch out loud and made them stand in a separate line. Everyone knew that if you received free lunch that you were too poor to pay for school lunch and probably received government assistance. Thankfully, things seem to have changed a lot over recent years and there is not as much shame and ridicule associated with receiving government assistance, but when I was growing up, other kids treated you like you had the plague when they found out that your family received assistance from the government.

My mother used to also make me walk to the store with empty soda bottles to cash in to receive a refund. I can remember when Pepsi soda came in an 8 pack of glass bottles. You would receive a deposit refund of $.10 for each empty bottle that you returned to the store. The neighborhood kids got a kick out of that when they saw me carrying multiple cases of empty bottles back to the store for a refund. The kids that saw me could not wait to get to school the next day to tell the other kids what they saw and that I was so poor that we did not have a car and had to walk to return those empty bottles for spare change.

I often had to go to school in clothes that were extremely outdated, pants with patches on the knees and that were too short which they called "high waters" back then and got bullied because of it. The bullying did not stop at being just verbal. Some kids would push me if I had to stand next to them in line or when the teacher told me to join their team at recess or in Physical Education (P.E.) class. They would knock my glasses off, pull my hair, hit me, kick me and spit on me because I was poor and couldn't afford nice brand name clothes and shoes. I believe my mom was trying to make life better for us by renting a small apartment in a decent neighborhood instead of moving us into a housing project in a high crime area, like she had grown up in. But I stuck out like a sore thumb at the schools I went to and was treated horribly.

Due to the teasing and bullying, when I got through middle school and went to high school, I stopped participating in any academic and extracurricular activities. I played basketball and ran track in middle school and part of my freshman year of high school. I loved running track and being part of a team, but the teasing and bullying continued there as well so I soon did not have any interest in participating. I started to skip classes my sophomore year of high school and this continued through my junior year. I withdrew from traditional high school at the beginning of my senior year and completed my studies for my high school diploma at an alternative learning center.

I did not just endure verbal and physical abuse at school. Verbal abuse was also a regular part of my home life. I believe that this was another example of a generational curse in our family. My mother had shared with me that her mother called her profane names when she was angry and she repeated that same behavior with me at times. It seemed like she may have favored my younger sister a little more and wasn't quite as mean to her. My little sister looked a lot like my mother. She had the same beautiful chocolate brown skin tone and features similar to my mother's.

My mother would often say that she was her little twin and did not fail to remind me that I looked just like my father and nothing like her. My mother was a victim of colorism due to her darker skin tone within her family and from others outside of her family. My maternal grandmother is Creole. She had a honey brown skin color and my maternal grandfather is Ethiopian. He had an espresso brown skin tone. All of my aunts had a light brown skin tone just a little darker than my grandmother's. My mother was the only one of my grandmother's children that had a dark skin tone that was similar to my grandfather's. My mother confessed that her mother often called her names and felt she treated her differently due to her darker skin tone. She said that other family members would often tease her and make derogatory statements about her due to her skin color. She shared that they often compared her to dark or black animals such as grizzly bears and gorillas. Colorism within our family was another generational issue we dealt with.

In addition to being raised by a young mother who struggled with mental health issues and alcohol use disorder, I believe that my mother was mean to me at times because of her upbringing, lack of support from my father and her financial situation. She also battled a mental health condition. I can recall my mother being diagnosed with depression and being prescribed medication. She took the medication a few times, said she did not like the way that they made her feel, and discontinued taking it. She was never a fan of modern medicine. She honestly did not like to take medicine of any kind.

She was a social drinker and would also consume alcohol when she was extremely stressed out. She always told me that alcohol use disorder was common on my father's side, but she did not have a problem with alcohol and could take it or leave it. However, I witnessed a substantial amount of alcohol consumption on my maternal side of my family as well. On a rare occasion, my mother would consume too much alcohol. With what I now know about alcohol use disorder, I would not have considered my mother an alcoholic or alcohol dependent, but at times she did use it to self-medicate, cope with her depression symptoms and to escape the memories of her past and her current situation. She did have an unhealthy relationship with alcohol because when she did drink, she would sometimes overindulge. Mental health issues and unhealthy relationships with alcohol are other examples of generational curses in our family.

Growing up I had no idea what a healthy relationship between a man and a woman looked like or what a "normal" or "traditional" family household consisted of. Whenever I went over to a friend's or a classmate's home, their families reminded me of the sitcoms I saw on TV shows like Growing Pains or the Cosby Show, because I didn't know any members of my family that had a family dynamic where the mother, father, siblings, and pets all lived together in one home happily ever after. My idea of relationships was based on what I saw in my family which was usually a single mother or a single mother with a significant other who argued, and sometimes physically fought. I believe that my mother saw the same scenarios play out in the generations before her.

My family does not consist of a bunch of "bad" people. Honestly, the members of my family are honest, caring and loving individuals. I believe that they were merely victims of their circumstances. They repeated the behaviors and actions of the generations that came before them and just did not know how or have the resources available to them to break the cycle. I believe that my generation and our offspring have broken these generational curses and tried to make better decisions so the generations to come will have a better quality of life, but we were damaged in the process of our upbringing. For me to move past the pain I endured from my upbringing, it required a lot of faith, prayer, understanding, compassion and forgiveness to shatter through this barrier and overcome this obstacle in my life. The following scripture helped me to overcome the pain and guilt that I had associated with my family's generational curses and continue to work to break them. Ezekiel 18:20 "The one who sins is the one who will die. The child will not share the guilt of the parent, nor will the parent share the guilt of the child. The righteousness of the righteous will be credited to them and the wickedness of the wicked will be charged against them."

CHAPTER
5

❀

ABANDONMENT/ LOSS

Aʙᴀɴᴅᴏɴᴍᴇɴᴛ ᴡᴀs ᴀɴᴏᴛʜᴇʀ ᴏʙsᴛᴀᴄʟᴇ ᴀɴᴅ ʙᴀʀʀɪᴇʀ ᴛʜᴀᴛ I ʜᴀᴅ ᴛᴏ shatter through. The earliest form of abandonment that I can remember came from my father. Although I was too young to remember, my mother told me that my father was abusive and struggled with alcohol use disorder. She stated that he would often spend his entire paycheck at the local bar getting intoxicated, forget that he had done so, accuse her of stealing the money and physically assault her.

My mother left my father when I was two years old and moved away from our hometown. After my mother left my father I could only remember seeing him one time when I was five years old and we had returned to our hometown to visit our family. Someone had told my father that we were in town and he said that he wanted to see me. He came to meet us at our relative's house. My mom and I were sitting in my aunt's car in front of the house. My mom was sitting in the front seat on the passenger's side of the car and I was sitting in the back seat directly behind her. I can recall when he approached the car, my mom rolled the window down about halfway and they talked for a couple of minutes.

Since I was only five years old and had not seen him since I was 2 years old, I did not recognize him. I had no idea who this man was talking to my mom. My mom eventually turned around in her seat and said, "Michelle, do you know who this is?" She was pointing out of the window in the direction of the tall man standing outside of my aunt's car. "I replied barely above a whisper, no." The tall man replied, "I'm your daddy." I had rolled my window down halfway when my mom rolled hers down to talk to my father, so I could hear everything that was going on.

My father stepped to the back of the car where I was sitting in the backseat and reached in and pulled me out of the car through the half rolled down window. He looked me directly in the face and said "Yeah, she's mine. She has my nose and my "good hair." He lifted me back through the window he had pulled me out of just a few minutes prior and told me that he loved me and would call me soon. I never heard from him again. The next time I heard about my father was when I was eight years old, and my mother told me one day when I had come home from school that he had a massive heart attack and passed away. He was only 36 years old.

She told me that she would not be attending the funeral and that she did not have any money to send me either. She would not allow me to go with anyone else to the funeral. She was very matter-of-factly and showed very little emotion. But, she had told me on many occasions that she hated my father for the way he treated her and I guess she hadn't forgiven him at that time. Other family members and friends of my father remember him as a hard working, kind and loving man.

To this day, I am not sure which is a more accurate description of who my father was as a man. What I do know is that the last memory that I have of him is the day I saw him in our hometown, and he told me he would call me and I never talked to him again. He also to my knowledge never sent a birthday card, wrote a letter or came to see me once he and my mother separated. After his statement that "yeah, she's mine", I wondered if the reason he never bothered to contact me or come see me was because he had some doubt about whether I was his biological child. Oddly enough, that thought made him not contacting me or coming to see me a little more palatable and gave me some comfort if that was his reasoning for being absent. Because I just do not understand someone having a child in the world and not wanting to at least check on them and see how they are doing. Even though I never had a relationship with my father, I surely missed his presence in my life. I unquestionably suffered from "daddy issues" from adolescence through my adult years.

There were also seasons in my life when I felt abandoned by my mother. Due to my less-than-optimal home life, and the cruelty I endured from other kids at school, I became distracted and began losing interest in going to school at a very rapid pace. I still possessed an unquenchable thirst for learning and knowledge, but it was exceptionally laborious to attempt to concentrate on schoolwork or pay attention in class when you were constantly having objects thrown at you, being spit on, pushed, kicked, hit, being teased, and talked about. I only had a couple of childhood friends and no one else I could really talk to.

Trying to navigate the already difficult and uncertain transition from my pubescent years to developing into a young woman, being what some would consider an outcast, having low self-esteem and basically no self-worth was a recipe for disaster. It was no surprise that I fell for the first smooth talking young man that showed me some attention and claimed he thought that I was pretty. He told me that he really liked me and it was love at first sight for him. He swiftly convinced me that if I felt the same way and wanted to be his girlfriend that I should prove it by engaging in sexual intercourse with him. He explained to me that us being intimate would solidify our relationship and affirm our love for each other.

I cannot say that my mother had not warned me about the lies that boys and men would tell to get what they wanted from a young lady. She had given me a version of the "birds and bees" talk. It went something like "I don't care what lies these guys tell you, these boys and men out here don't want anything from you besides sex. If you know what is good for you, you better keep your head down, in those books and make something out of yourself because if you mess around out in these streets and get pregnant, you are going to be looking for a new place to live because I am not raising any more kids. I can barely feed, clothe and keep a roof over your heads." But what this young man was telling me was different. He seemed honest enough. He was nice to me. I had fooled myself into believing that he truly liked me for my brains and personality. So, I let down my guard and gave in to his persuasion.

A couple of months after my "boyfriend" and I were intimate, my mom asked me one day if I needed any feminine products. I told her that I did not need anymore and still had plenty left. She asked me how I had plenty left when she had not bought me any in several months. Before I could answer her first question, she asked me when my last menstrual cycle was. I shrugged my shoulders and told her that I wasn't sure and that I could not remember. She asked me if I was still writing it on the calendar like she had told me to when I first started my menstrual cycle, so that I would have an idea when it was coming each month and not be caught off guard and unprepared at school. I told her yes, I was. She started thumbing through the calendar that hung on the wall between the kitchenette and living area of our apartment. I continued doing what I was doing before she asked me the question because I couldn't understand why she was so concerned with my menstrual cycle all of a sudden. Her voice roared like thunder when she said, "You haven't had a cycle in three months!" Her voice startled me out of whatever daydream I was in. Now that she had mentioned it, it had been a long time since I had a menstrual cycle.

She took me to Planned Parenthood the very next day and a nurse confirmed that I was about 8 weeks pregnant. The nurse asked me if I had used any birth control or protection. I shook my head, no. She started handing me multiple pamphlets and explaining what my options were. I didn't hear much of what she said after that. I was speechless and in complete shock. I glanced out of the corner of my eye and saw that my mother was silently crying. When the nurse stepped out of the room, I put my hand on my mother's and asked if she was ok? She immediately pulled her hand back and said "You have no idea what you have done. You are only 15 years old. You messed up your life girl!" After we left the clinic, my mother was eerily quiet for the rest of the evening. She moved through her nightly routine of cooking, washing the dishes (this was usually my chore, so I knew something was wrong because she did them and did not say a word), watching her game shows, taking a bath and going to bed about 9:00 PM.

When I woke up the next morning to get ready for school, she was sitting on the couch with her back to me looking out of the window. We lived in a 3rd floor apartment. She often sat and looked out the window, staring up at the sky when there was something weighing heavily on her mind. Once I was completely ready for school and heading out the door, I said like I always did, "Bye, Mama. Have a nice day." She replied, without ever turning around to look at me, "While you are at school today, I want you to think about where you are going to stay because like I told you, if you ever get pregnant, you can't stay here. I can't afford another mouth to feed." As usual, when my feelings were hurt, I could feel the tears welling up in my eyes as I shut the front door behind me.

My mother followed through on her threat and when I returned home from school that day, most of my clothes and belongings were packed up in bags. I had no idea where I was going to go. I only had a couple of friends. I could ask one of them if I could spend a couple of nights at their house. However, during my teenage years, parents called each other to make sure that you had permission from your parents before allowing someone to stay at their house. I knew my mother. As soon as they called her, she was going to tell them everything and those parents would not want me at their house.

My "boyfriend" said that his mother worked a 2nd and 3rd shift job, and I could stay over there on the days that she worked. So, I stayed the night at his house on the days that his mother worked. On the days that she did not work I tried to sneak and crash at one of my friend's houses. On the nights that my "boyfriend's" mother did not work and one of my friends could not sneak me in to crash at their house, I would sleep in the back of my mother's friend's pickup truck. It was a small pickup truck with a camper shell. He was an older, retired gentleman that lived in the same apartment building that we did. My mother did not drive, and he often drove her around to run errands. Because I had rode along with them on many occasions, I knew that he never locked the camper shell on his truck. I also knew that he usually never left his apartment after 9:00 PM. If I was up and out of the back of that camper by 7:00 AM no one would know I was sleeping in there.

The rotating between sleeping at my "boyfriend's" house, my friend's house and the back of my mother's boyfriend's truck went on for several weeks. I have always been an organized person, so it was killing me to live this way, with no real place to call home. I guess some would call it a blessing in disguise or God's will, but I ended up having a miscarriage at about 14 weeks. My mother eventually allowed me to return home but did not let me forget how I had disappointed her and how ashamed of me she was. This was a season in my life where I felt abandoned on an entirely different level. I was so embarrassed that I had let this happen that I couldn't even talk to my sister about how I was feeling.

My sister was still in the military during this time and doing well for herself. My mother had already told my sister her version of what was going on with me, which was that I was "wild and out of control." This could not have been further from the truth. I was still the same shy, quiet, timid, girl with low self-esteem who I always was. I assumed that even though my sister had lived under my mother's roof and knew firsthand how difficult my mother could be that she must have believed the things that she told her, because I didn't get as many letters from her as before the situation happened and my mother stop telling me that my sister wanted to talk to me when she called (when my sister and I discussed this later on down the line, we discovered that my mother was also telling my sister that I did not want to talk to her because I was too caught up in the boy who had gotten me pregnant).

I was none of those things that she described to my sister. I was just a 15-year-old girl, who still read the Babysitters Club Books by Ann M. Martin and the Ramona book collection by

Beverly Cleary looking for a way to fit in with other teenagers my age, be accepted and looking for a way to stop the pain, even if it was just temporarily. This situation again evinced what I already knew, which was that my mother could not give me what she didn't acquire from her mother in her upbringing. Her mother talked and treated her in the same manner that she talked to and treated me. For me to shatter through this barrier and overcome this obstacle, I had to ask for God's help and guidance in teaching me how to forgive myself for sinning and engaging in intercourse before marriage, forgive my mother, for her lack of empathy, hardheartedness, and putting me out in the world to fend for myself in one of my darkest hours and ask Him to help me learn how to avoid treating others, including my children, the way that I was treated. (Psalm 27:10-14-"Though my father and mother forsake me, the Lord will receive me. Teach me your way Lord; lead me in a straight path because of my oppressors. Do not turn me over to the desire of my foes, for false witnesses rise up against me, spouting malicious accusations. I remain confident of this; I will see the goodness of the Lord in the land of the living. Wait for the Lord; be strong and take heart and wait for the Lord.")

I also felt abandoned by my mother later in life when she passed away. Despite the strained relationship that my mother and I had during my childhood and teenage years, we became extremely close when I became a mother. The saying "There is no handbook for raising children" made so much more sense to me after I had my own children. I began to more clearly understand the struggles that she faced being a single mother, with an intellectual disability, mental health issues, living at poverty level and having a challenging and less than ideal upbringing. Instead of holding those things against her I began to admire her strength to persevere and try to give us what she did not have. I wanted my children to have a close relationship with their grandmother so I made the extra effort to ensure that our bond was tight. My mom began to experience health issues in her early 40's. She had gestational diabetes when she was pregnant with my younger sister in her mid 30's. She was later diagnosed with Type 2 diabetes. Much like her attitude towards her mental health and wellness, my mother did not follow the doctor's advice and continued to eat an unhealthy diet, stress and live a sedentary lifestyle. Her condition worsened. She became insulin dependent and had to inject herself with her diabetes medication multiple times daily. A few years later she was diagnosed with congestive heart failure and eventually had to have quadruple bypass heart surgery.

After the heart surgery, her doctors warned that if she wanted to live a full life that she would have to change her lifestyle. She tried for a little while, but eventually resumed her previous habits which eventually led to her death nine years after having heart surgery. She moved in with me during the last year of her life and developed an extremely close relationship with all of my kids, who were all teenagers at the time. She truly suffered the last couple of months of her life. Losing her was devastating for the entire family. I felt abandoned by her because she was a huge part of my life. Even though she wasn't the most compassionate and empathetic mother, I knew that she loved me and I had never navigated this world without her. I could not fathom why she did not fight harder to change her lifestyle so she could live a longer life, be here for her kids and to see her grandchildren and great grandchildren grow up. Losing my father at the age of 36 and my mother at 63, made me passionate about doing everything within my power to live a healthier lifestyle and help others do the same. Hopefully by living a healthier lifestyle, I can prevent my kids from enduring the same pain that I did by losing a parent prematurely.

CHAPTER
6

❁

SELF-IMAGE/
SELF LOVE

From as far back as I can remember I have struggled with my self-image and self-esteem. My poor self-image and low self-esteem eventually began to affect my self-worth and self-love. I can recall my mother laughing and telling me at a very young age that the first thing that my grandmother said about me when she saw me was that my nose was wide and was spread all over my face just like the rest of my dad's family. She advised my mother to put a wooden clothes pin on my nose at night while I slept to reshape my nose while I was still a baby, before it "got out of control" and negatively impacted my looks. My mother said that she told my grandmother that she wasn't going to do that to her baby, but I still found it hurtful that this was the first thing my grandmother said about me when she saw me and the fact that my mother found her suggestion humorous.

I continued to receive those types of negative comments from my grandmother whenever I saw her. She told me that she was glad that I was smart because I wasn't much to look at. She said that I could probably find and keep a husband if I learned to be submissive enough and a good wife. I knew that my grandmother indulged in alcohol on a regular basis, so I thought she made a lot of those negative and hurtful comments because she was under the influence. When we later discovered that she was battling a mental health condition these comments made more sense. This discovery made her making these inappropriate comments more understandable, but did not make them sting any less.

My mother used to also make jokes about me wearing glasses, having impaired vision and being clumsy. She said I reminded her of Mr. Magoo, who was a cartoon character from the 1960's because we both wore thick eyeglasses. I was born with a condition called strabismus, which is an eye muscle disorder which causes poor eye muscle control and the eyes do not always look in the same direction and at the same time. Some people also refer to this condition as having "crossed eyes" or being "cockeyed." I had to start wearing glasses before the age of 1 to try to strengthen my eye muscles and align my eyes to look in the same direction at the same time. That treatment method was not successful, and I had to undergo my first eye surgery at the age of five. That procedure helped my condition cosmetically for several years, but as I approached my pre-teen years, the muscles in my right eye became weak and my eyes were becoming unaligned again. I underwent another surgery in my early 30s in an attempt to cosmetically correct this condition again. My eye condition was another reason that I was teased and bullied a lot in school. I think that my mother believed that she was being funny and making light of the situation to make me feel better and to not take the teasing I received at school so seriously, but it actually hurt my feelings. Because she was my mom, her words weighed heavily and influenced my self-esteem.

My grandfather (my grandmother's ex husband) also gave me the nickname "tangle foot" because I was extremely "pigeon-toed." He would say "My goodness girl everything is crossed up on you, your eyes and your feet. Go ahead and sit down somewhere before you trip over your own feet and turn something over in here." Again, I don't think he was intentionally being cruel or insensitive to my conditions, but his words really hurt my feelings. He had cute little nicknames for his other granddaughters like "Baby girl", "Angel" and "Genie", but his nickname for me reminded me of conditions that I constantly got teased about and had no control over. I have heard this type of taunting and teasing going on in other families as well. When I got older and heard family members or friends making fun of each other's differences such as weight, skin tone or facial features, I would let them know that their words may not be funny to the person they are directed at and they may hurt the other person's feelings. I would often get responses like "Aww, they know I love them" or "I am just playing with them." I could never understand why this type of behavior was okay or why people who claimed to love each other would talk to each other that way even if they were just playing around.

Several years ago, I visited my hometown and stopped by to see a relative whom I had not seen in over 30 years and had recently reconnected with on Facebook. One of the first things she said to me was "Girl you are wider than all outside, just like your mama was. She was just a lot darker than you." I could not believe she felt comfortable saying those words to me, not only because she hadn't seen me in over 30 years and barely knew me, but also out of respect for my mother who had just passed away a few months prior to my visit there. I am often shocked at the lack of regard some family members have for each other and just say the first thing that comes to their mind. I don't know if she felt this was acceptable to say to me because she was my elder, but it wasn't. We need to be more mindful of the things that we say to each other. It is not okay to talk negatively about and belittle others, regardless if they are family or not.

I was also teased about the way that I spoke. I was often asked why I was always trying to "speak so proper or sound like I was White." I did not understand why or how they had come to that conclusion. I used standard grammar and spoke proper English. By the time I had reached adulthood I was self-conscious about my eyes, glasses, skin, feet, weight, the way I spoke and the fact that I had gotten pregnant as a teenager. I got teased about many of these things from other students at school, but it was even more painful, when relatives said cruel things and threw up my past or my flaws in my face.

The mean words and vile jokes over the years about my nose and appearance had wreaked havoc on my self-esteem. The negative comments about my nose and looks in general had been embedded in my psyche since I was a young child. I began to hate the way that I looked. I used to spend a lot of time in the mirror at school and home trying to apply make-up and make sure my hair was perfect to improve my looks. Some family members and people would tease me about that also. As a result of having a bad case of acne as a teenager, and having a nervous habit of picking at my face when I was feeling anxious, I had a lot of scarring and dark marks on my face. I would apply an excessive amount of makeup to try and hide the scarring. Of course, people assumed that I was wearing so much makeup to look older and attract men, when I was truthfully trying to create the illusion that I had clear skin, but failed miserably at that attempt.

I can remember like it was yesterday overhearing someone who I worked with at a fast-food restaurant as a teenager tell another co-worker that I had so much makeup on that I looked like a corpse. They started laughing loudly and pointing in my direction causing a disruption in the dining area of the restaurant. As soon as I finished helping the customer who was standing at my register the entire time this was going on, I advised my supervisor that I wasn't feeling well and needed to go home immediately. Even though I really liked working there and needed the extra money, I was so humiliated by what my co-worker had said that I caught the city bus home that day and never returned to that job. Although I truly believed in my heart that I was a loving, caring, kind, empathetic, hard-working, intelligent person with a good heart, my overall self-image was poor, and my self-worth was non-existent. I allowed people to talk to me and about me in any kind of way they pleased. I basically gave them permission to run all over me by not speaking up for myself. I just did not have that fight in me, know how to kill them with kindness, or slay them with the word of God back then. It seemed like the few times that I did try to stand up for myself, the situation just escalated, and the outcome was worse than when I remained quiet and tried to ignore it.

I started to become extremely withdrawn and depressed. I experienced intense anxiety symptoms when I was around groups of people. I rarely left the house except for school or work. I was just exhausted with everything and did not see any relief in sight. On the rare occasion that I shared some of what I was going through with someone, they would usually insinuate that I was overreacting, that everyone dealt with being talked about and I just needed to grow a thicker skin. They would make it seem like they were just so strong, in control, and that they didn't let little things like that bother them. But the more I looked at their behavior I noticed that they were mean at times and lashed out at others. It wasn't that they were so strong, they just took their pain and anger out on other people. That was their release, and I did not have a release, I was holding all my pain and anger inside. I did not want to start taking my anger and pain out on others becoming part of the problem instead of being part of the solution. I say all this to say that we need to be more mindful, caring, and compassionate with our words and interactions with others. We never know what other people are going through or dealing with. The two scriptures that have helped me tame my tongue are Proverbs 18:21 "The tongue has the power of life and death, and those who love it will eat its fruit." James 3:9 "With the tongue we praise our Lord and Father, and with it we curse human beings, who have been made in God's likeness."

The teasing and ridicule did not stop when I became an adult. I was not getting physically bullied but some people still felt that it was okay to say whatever crossed their mind to me. I believe that they could tell that I was shy and timid because I often unintentionally held my head down during interactions and was usually very quiet; only speaking when being spoken to. People often said things about my weight like "wow girl you really blew up since high school" or "I almost didn't recognize you with all of the weight that you gained" to me as calmly as if they were asking me if I would like a stick of gum. As many times as people have made these unsolicited obnoxious comments to me, I was always caught off guard by them and totally unprepared to respond.

Comments like these have also been directed at me from people that I barely know. One day I was giving a presentation about a project that I had been selected to oversee and manage. The presentation was flawless and I was extremely proud of all of the hard work that I had put into it. Most of the people who were in attendance at the meeting gave me kudos and high praises for the detail, information and knowledge that I shared with them. However, I heard one meeting attendee make the statement "I do not know how she is going to manage a multi-million dollar project when she can't manage to put her fork down." Of course the other couple of people that he was talking to found his comment amusing. I learned two very important things from that incident (1) some people are always going to judge you solely on your outer appearance and (2) there was definitely such a thing as weight prejudice and discrimination, even in the workplace. I have been in a toxic relationship where someone has made a disparaging remark about my weight or size as soon as they became angry. However, this was the first time, (but definitely not the last time) that I witnessed this behavior in the workplace.

In addition to the cosmetic surgery that I had performed to correct my eye condition, I eventually also opted to have rhinoplasty surgery or more commonly known as a "nose job." It breaks my heart when I see people bashing others for having cosmetic surgery to alter or enhance their appearance. Yes, some of the people that have these procedures may be doing it for vanity reasons, but many of them are doing it because they are self-conscience about their face and/or body, because of the hurtful things that have been said to them or about their appearance and it has impacted their self-esteem, self- image, and self-worth. Having the cosmetic surgery did aid me in feeling better about my appearance, but praying to God and having faith in His word helped to improve my self-image, gain self-worth and increase my self-confidence. I now have authentic self-love, hope, joy and I have started showing off the one trait that I did receive many compliments on throughout my life which is my smile. There is a quote that I heard many years ago and I keep it near and dear to my heart because it is so true and I had to learn to apply it to my everyday life. "Let your smile change the world. Don't let the world change your smile." I had to start looking at and seeing myself and others through God's eyes instead of human eyes in order to shatter through this barrier and overcome the obstacle of low self-esteem, poor self-image and non-existent self-worth. The following scripture helped me achieve genuine self-love and appreciation. (Psalm 139:13-14 "For you created my inmost being. You knit me together in my mother's womb. I praise you because I am fearfully and wonderfully made; your works are wonderful. I know that full well") .

CHAPTER
7

❀

OVERCOMING TRAUMA

TRAUMA AND ABUSE WERE OTHER BARRIERS THAT I HAD TO SHATTER through in my life to become the best version of me. I believe that the abuse that I tolerated was directly related to the violence that I witnessed as a child in addition to having low self-esteem. Since I witnessed physical altercations as a child it did not seem completely foreign to me when my first "boyfriend" assaulted me when I was 15 years old. He had grabbed my arm a little too tightly, pushed and shoved me a couple of times prior to that incident when he did not like something I said, did or an outfit I wore, which startled and frightened me. But he always told me afterwards that he was just playing around with me and he would never actually harm me.

The first time it happened was a couple of days after I had the miscarriage. He wanted to be intimate and I very honestly told him that I had a lot on my mind and was not interested. I didn't feel physically well after the ordeal my body had just gone through. I was struggling to concentrate in school and my grades were beginning to suffer. I could tell by the expression on his face that he did not understand or just did not care about what I was going through.

He was a couple of years older than me and was always skipping school so he definitely could not relate to my concerns about my grades. His advice was that since I would be 16 soon and could legally drop out at that age and take the high school equivalency exam to obtain my G.E.D. certificate that I shouldn't be concerned with my grades. He kept trying to touch me and coerce me into laying down across his bed. I kept resisting and moving his hands. He became a little more forceful in trying to push me down and get on top of me. I eventually told him that I was going to leave and go to my friend's house. He jumped up and stood in front of his bedroom door, preventing me from being able to leave. He asked me what my problem was. I told him again that I was not in the mood and was not feeling very well. He said that he didn't believe that was all that was going on. He said that he noticed that I had been dressing differently when I went to school and I hadn't been coming over to his house as much. I explained that since I now had a part-time job, I could buy nicer clothes and since I was working and going to school, I did not have as much spare time to come over to his house.

He went on to say that if I wasn't interested in being intimate with him then I must be seeing someone else. He continued on with his rant saying that if I didn't give him what he wanted, then he would find another girl who would. At this point, I had realized that I really didn't like him as much as I thought. Staying over his house a few nights a week when his mother worked a double shift allowed me to see that he was very aggressive, smoked, drank alcohol, and was very flirtatious and inappropriate with any other females who came over to visit anyone that lived in the home. Also after the whole pregnancy situation, getting told to leave my mother's home, my grade slipping and how much guilt and shame I felt for sinning against God in the first place, I realized what a big mistake I made and wanted to get out of the situation. But since I wasn't able to return home yet, I didn't have many options at the time.

I guess he had said something to me that I didn't hear or respond to because the next thing I knew he grabbed me by my throat and said "So now you don't hear me talking to you?" His hand was so tight around my neck that when I tried to respond, nothing came out. "Oh you think I am a joke? I am going to show you that I am nothing to play with." He threw me down on his bed and immediately dove on top of me and proceeded to try to hold me down with one arm and try to get my sundress up with his free hand. We tussled for what seemed like forever. Tears were welling up in my eyes, but he wouldn't stop. We were both sweating and out of breath. I asked what he was doing and pleaded with him to stop, but he just kept saying that he could show me better than he could tell me.

I had heard about these types of things happening to other girls and women, but I could not believe that this was happening and especially with someone who was supposed to be my "boyfriend." The word rape or sexual assault did not immediately come to mind. I just knew I felt like what was happening was really wrong and that I was being violated. When I refused to stop resisting, he grabbed a fistful of my hair and snatched my head back. He was gritting his teeth and when I finally looked up at him his eyes looked like he was staring right through me. His facial expression looked very hateful and deranged.

I was sobbing by this point and still trying to get away from his grip with the little strength that I had left. "Oh so you're still not going to give me what I want?" he said. Before, I could even respond, he opened his mouth and bit me on my shoulder really hard. He continued to slowly penetrate his teeth deeper into my skin until I stopped struggling because the pain from the bite was so intense. After holding the bite for what seemed like a couple of minutes at least, he finally stopped biting me and asked me if I was going to act right now. I was speechless. I just laid there motionless. I did not say a word as he forced himself on me. I always had a vivid imagination. I remember imagining I was somewhere else until he was finished. When he was done, I slowly got up off the bed. I tried to brush my hair down with my hand and proceeded to exit his bedroom.

He said in a calm voice "Hey you coming back over later when you leave your friend's house?" I looked at him over my shoulder in shock. He did not look hateful and deranged anymore. He looked disturbingly calm and relaxed especially considering what had just taken place. I just shook my head no and left. This situation seemed different from the stories I had heard from other women. This wasn't a stranger or acquaintance that had viciously forced himself on me. This was someone who was not much older than me, who had said that he loved me, someone I had lost my virginity to and someone that I thought I cared deeply for. But this was still sexual assault because the act was not consensual.

That incident was the first time that I experienced trauma at the hands of someone that I was dating, but it wasn't the last. The next time that I was physically assaulted was a couple of years after the first incident occurred, and I had been dating someone else for several months. It seemed to be going really well. He was the complete opposite of the first guy that I dated. He was several years older than me, in college, had a steady job and seemed like the perfect gentleman. He always spoke to me in a soft and kind tone. He always answered my mom with a yes ma'am or no ma'am and appeared to be a well-rounded, respectful person.

It was Valentine's Day. He had come to pick me up to go on a date. I wasn't quite ready when he got there, so he came inside to continue to wait for me to finish getting ready. My mother was in her bedroom which was located in the rear of the apartment with the TV blaring. My bedroom was in the front of the apartment. When I let him in, he followed me back to my bedroom and sat on the edge of the bed and handed me the bag that he was carrying and said "Happy Valentine's Day '' with a wide grin on his face. I smiled back and said thank you and handed him the gift that I had gotten for him. I sat the bag on the edge of my bed and lifted out a small box and placed it on the bed next to the bag and reached back in the bag to grab the card out when I realized there were actually two cards in the bag. On the front of one of the cards, I saw my name. The other card had a female name that I did not recognize. I held up the card and asked, "Who is this card for? "The smile that had just been spread across his face quickly disappeared. He hesitated a long while before responding "Oh that's nothing. That card is for one of my close friends." He began to fidget with the keys in his pocket and look around the room nervously.

I started to open the flap of the envelope to see what had been written inside of the card because I thought that I had met most of his friends. I had never heard him mention this "close friend's" name before. He quickly snatched the envelope out of my hands and asked me in a stern tone "What do you think you are doing?" I responded, "I want to see what is written on the card, because I have never heard you mention that name before." He looked extremely irritated and said "I don't have to prove anything to you. Stop acting so insecure. I have a lot of female friends that you don't know. You haven't met everybody that I know." I tried to grab the envelope from his hands again. He pushed me back and held the envelope just out of my reach. When he pushed me, I was caught off guard, lost my balance and fell on the floor. He didn't bother to try to help me to my feet. He just stood over me and said "Look at you acting ignorant and being dramatic. Get up girl. I barely touched you."

I continued to sit on the floor for a few seconds looking up at him with what I am sure was a confused expression on my face. This behavior was nothing like him. He had always been so nice, kind and courteous towards me. He had never even raised his voice when speaking to me. He just stared at me with a look of disgust on his face. As I picked myself up off of the floor, I said "I want to see what you wrote on the card?" He said, "You aren't going to see anything!" as he tore the card into small pieces. "If she was just a friend, why didn't you let me see what was on the card?" "Because it wasn't any of your business, that's why." At that point, I was furious and told him that I was no longer in the mood to go out with him and he should just leave. I started towards the front door so I could let him out.

He snatched me back by my arm and asked in an angry tone, "So you are going to cancel our plans because I bought my friend a card?" I told him that I did not feel like discussing it and I was tired and just going to go to bed. He started poking me in the forehead with his finger and said, "If I leave tonight, we are done. I responded in a calm tone. "Okay, that's fine. If you are buying someone else a card for Valentine's Day, we are already done." I didn't even see the punch coming and just felt his fist connect with my cheekbone and the blows kept coming all over my face and head after that. I was so caught off guard, and his hands were moving so fast, that all I could do was try to shield my face before the next punch landed. The blows came to an abrupt stop and he said "Man, what am I doing. I am so sorry. I didn't mean to do that. Are you okay?" I just stood there trembling and touching my face and head to see if I was bleeding from anywhere because my face and head were throbbing.

I had almost forgotten that my mom was back in her bedroom watching TV. Lord, if she knew this man was in her house hitting her daughter, I don't know what she might do. He was still apologizing and was now sitting on the edge of my bed with his head in his hands rocking back and forth repeating "Man, I am sorry. I am really sorry. You know I didn't mean to do that."

My head and face were both hurting in multiple areas and it felt like my right cheek bone was rapidly swelling. I asked him to leave again. He replied, "I can't leave until you say that you forgive me and that we are going to work this out." I would have said anything to get him out of that house. I heard my mother stirring around in her bedroom. I could not let her see me like this, especially when he was still in her house. I told him "Yeah I forgive you and we can work it out." I would have said just about anything at that moment to get him out of that house. I wish I could say that I stopped seeing him immediately after that incident happened. But I did not and there were several other violent incidents after that one. The worst attack left me with my bottom lip split open and a black eye that was swollen shut. But after many nights of prayer and soul searching, I did get out of that violent relationship.

These were a few of the examples of the abuse and trauma I have endured throughout my life. It was scary and painful at the time. I had no clue how serious and dangerous these situations were until much later on because I witnessed this type of behavior as a child growing up and I had normalized it in my mind. I was always baffled at how quickly a person could change or reveal their true colors and go from being someone that you trusted to being someone who you feared because they were violating you. There was one other incident that happened prior to those that involved someone who we considered a family friend.

My mother used to like to sometimes invite friends from the neighborhood over to our apartment on the weekends to play cards. She would cook food and tell me that I was in charge of the music and drinks, which basically meant I would be expected to stay within earshot and play whatever music they wanted to hear and run to the refrigerator to get cold drinks whenever someone told me to. Most of the people that she invited over either lived in our building or on the same street that we did. Sometimes someone at these card parties would have too much to drink and she would allow them to lay down on the couch in an attempt to sleep off the effects.

One day, one of the guys who often came to these parties showed up to the party late and already visibly intoxicated. Most of the neighbors and friends who had attended the card party had already left. There was just my mom and a couple of other people remaining in our apartment when he showed up. He was staggering and his speech was very slurred. He almost fell on my mother, who was still sitting at the card table, when he tried to give her a hug. My mother who was never one to hold her tongue said "You are sloppy drunk. Go lay down on the couch and sleep it off." He tried to protest but there was no winning when it came to debating with my mom. She got up from her seat at the table and led him over to the couch. He mumbled something and then ended up falling asleep sitting straight up.

My mother told me she and the couple of the people remaining at the card party were going to the store and that she would be right back. She told me to warm up some soup to give to her friend who was asleep on the couch in case he woke up and to keep an eye on my younger sister. I took a pot out of the cabinet to warm up some soup like my mother had told me to. My younger sister was back in my mother's bedroom watching TV. I could hear her laughing at whatever she was watching every now and again. After I had finished warming up the soup and put it in a bowl and placed it in the oven, I tried to turn around from the stove to head back into my bedroom. But, when I attempted to turn around, I bumped into my mom's friend who had apparently been woken up by the noise I was making in the kitchenette trying to warm up the soup and was now standing directly behind me. He was rocking back and forth and not steady on his feet. I quickly took a couple of side steps to put some distance between us.

He leaned over almost losing his balance and put his hand on my shoulder and slurred "About how old are you now? I know you have a boyfriend. I can tell by the way that you are filling out those pants." He stood there looking me up and down and licking his lips. I was disgusted by the way this much older man who was supposed to be my mother's friend was looking at me but I just ignored his question because I knew he was drunk and probably had no idea who I was or what he was saying at that moment. I tried to quickly change the subject by saying, "If you want to sit at the table, I can bring you some soup. Mama told me to make it for you. She should be back any minute." He came closer to me and put his arm around my neck. I cringed when he touched me and quickly backed away from him. His clothes and breath reeked of alcohol.

I was still trying to be respectful and ignore his advances because my mother considered him a friend, he was my elder and I had seen on many occasions how alcohol could make someone act out of character. I grabbed the soup out of the oven and put it on the card table that was sitting in the middle of our living area and said "Come and sit down and eat some of this soup." He swung his hand in the direction of the soup sitting on the table in what I believe was an attempt to knock it off the table, but he was so intoxicated that his aim was off and missed hitting the bowl of soup. He yelled, "I don't want no soup. I want you girl." He took several quick steps towards me and was sticking his tongue out making weird moaning noises. He reached out and touched me inappropriately. I roughly pushed his hands away. He reached in his pocket and pulled out a crumpled up five dollar bill and tried to hand it to me. I did not reach for the money and took a few more steps back, not taking my eyes off of him. He said, slurring every other word, "Here girl. You better take this money. I know your mama is strict on you and doesn't give you any money. Here, take it."

I knew I needed to get myself and my sister out of that apartment. I backed out of the living area of our apartment leaving him standing there rambling, looking me up and down with his bloodshot eyes and still holding that raggedy five dollar bill in his hand, shaking it at me. I rushed back to my mom's room where my sister was still watching TV. Even though it was the middle of winter and snowing outside, I picked her up and put her on my hip and rushed out the front door of our apartment. My sister was about five years old at the time and asking a thousand questions about why we were leaving our apartment, where we were going, and why we didn't put our coats on. We lived on the top floor of the apartment building that had a back fire escape. I sat on that back fire escape holding my little sister on my lap and trying to answer her questions without alarming her that anything was wrong. I did not want her to feel frightened like I had at times during my childhood.

I could still hear my mother's friend stumbling around in our apartment and calling out to me every few minutes. I tried to imagine what my older sister would do in this situation. I knew that she would have tried to make me feel safe even though she was scared herself and she would do everything in her power to make sure that she kept me safe. I guess I had gotten lost in my own thoughts and imagination as I often did when reality became too painful for me to bear, because I heard my little sister's tiny voice calling my name, "Chelle, I want to go back in the house, it is cold out here. I want to watch TV." I had grabbed my sister so fast and ran out of the house, I hadn't had time to grab her or myself a coat or jacket. I had on a short sleeved top and a pair of blue jeans and my little sister had on a pair of the onesie pajamas that had the feet in them and zipped up in the front.

I squeezed her a little tighter to try to warm her up and told her that we could go back in the house soon, but right now we were playing a fun game. I explained to her that we were on an important mission and we had to hide from our mother's friend who could still be heard fumbling around in our apartment. I told her that the fire escape was our secret and magical hiding spot. I went on to tell her that we were invisible and safe as long as we stayed on the fire escape, but we had to try to be very quiet so that he couldn't hear us and that we could hear our mother's voice when she got back from the store because she was on our team and would rescue us.

My little sister had no clue that we were really out in the freezing cold hiding from my mom's friend because he was inebriated and had tried to assault me and at that point she didn't need to know. All she needed to do was be a five-year old kid. She giggled with excitement and rubbed her little hands together and said "Ok, Chelle. This is fun. I can be really quiet. We are going to win this game!" I heard footsteps coming up the front stairs of our apartment and my mother's voice talking and laughing with her friends. My little sister screeched, "Mama is back Chelle. She can save us now. We won the game!"

My sister tried to pull open the door to the fire escape but it was too heavy for her, so I helped her open it and she rushed in. Before I could even walk through the fire escape door behind my little sister, my mother was glaring at me with her hands on her hips and yelled, "Where have y'all been? And why do you have my baby outside with no coat on? My little sister tried to tell her about the game, but she instantly told her to be quiet and to go back to her bedroom to watch TV. She continued to glare at me. "I'm waiting for an answer."

The people who had taken my mother to the store were now drinking the beverages that they had bought talking and laughing with my mother's friend who seemed to have sobered up a bit and talking more clearly. I told my mother what transpired while she was at the store. I knew that my mother had a few drinks and did not want her to make a scene or get into an altercation with her friend over what happened, so I told her in a very low voice that when she left he woke up, started talking weird and tried to grab me, so I took my sister and went on the fire escape to wait for her to get back.

My mother shouted, "So you're telling me he tried to attack you?" It seemed like everyone stopped talking at once and was staring at my mother and I. You could hear a pin drop. My mom rushed over to her friend who was sitting on the couch, pointed her finger in his face and asked, "Did you touch my daughter?" He leaned his head back, chuckled a little and said "Nah, you know me better than that. I just gave her a little money for making me the soup and she just snatched it and walked off." I could not believe that this man was sitting there telling that barefaced lie. "Mama, he is lying!" I screamed.

"Girl, who are you hollering at and you know better than to call a grown person a liar. And what did I tell you about asking and accepting money from grown men? You are way too old for that now. You are at the age where if you ask them for something, they are going to surely ask you for something. You know you know better. I told you that a long time ago." She continued on ranting and raving, but seemed to be talking more to herself than to me at this point. She told him to get out of her house and not to come back.

I fought back the tears, accepted the situation because I knew that nothing I said or did at that point would make a difference now and tried to put the experience out of my mind, but what I really did was stuff it down inside me like I had done with all of my other pain, abuse and trauma. I prayed to God that even though I had not been shown empathy, compassion, and love in the way that I needed it, that He would show me how to exhibit love to my children, family and to others in the way that they needed it. I did not pray for Him to show me how to exhibit compassion and empathy. It seemed like I was born innately knowing how to show empathy and compassion for others, even those who had hurt me.

My family and friends always teased me about having a bleeding heart. I tried to love, help, and see the good in everybody.

I would even cry when sad things happened on TV or a movie. They would say, "Girl you know this is fake and those are actors right?" I would calmly reply, "Yeah, but these shows and movies are based on real life and things like that really happen in our world every day and I think it's sad" They would just laugh at me. I used to dislike the fact that I cried at the drop of a dime and wore my feelings on my sleeve. I later learned that being empathetic and compassionate were gifts from God. It allowed me to put myself in other people's shoes and have the ability to forgive and help others.

I prayed to God that he would give me the strength and understanding to forgive my mother's friend for trying to assault me and lying to my mother about what happened. God answered my prayers as he always did. I mentioned earlier in this book that God can reveal a message or an answer to your prayers through mysterious methods and sources, even through "secular" content. So you want to ensure that your mind and heart is open to receive them.

One day, I was watching the show Law and Order, SVU. I honestly never understood why I was always drawn to watch this show because it was about detectives trying to solve sexual crimes. I usually did not like to watch shows like that and usually opted to watch more feel good movies and comedies. But for some reason, if I flipped through the channels and it was on, I would always watch it. This episode showed a scene where an intoxicated man was trying to grope and assault a teenage girl. He was trying to coerce her into having intercourse by promising to give her money and gifts. Of course, it triggered me to think back to the experience that I had with my mother's friend.

When I went to sleep that night, I had a dream about that episode of Law and Order SVU. The scene looked the same as in the episode that I had seen earlier. However, when I took a closer look it was me and my mother's friend in the scene instead of the actors that I saw earlier on the show. I rubbed my eyes in the dream to make sure I was actually seeing what I thought I was seeing and when I looked back at the man, his face now looked exactly like my son's. I rubbed my eyes again and looked up as the man started to disappear and a huge projector screen appeared in the area where he was standing before. It began to flash through scenes of what looked like an old movie starring my mother's friend who had tried to assault me many years before.

I interpreted the scenes as a reflection of different periods in my mother's friend's life. The different scenes showed him as a baby, as a small child getting physically bullied and abused, him passing out food and supplies to people in our neighborhood, him going into the military and having a friend die in his arms, him at his mother's funeral leaning over her casket weeping, and him drinking bottles and bottles of liquor one after the other. Then the movie abruptly stopped. The exceptionally eerie part was that throughout the dream, his face was constantly changing. In some of the scenes in the dream his face looked like his own and then morphed into my son's face and in other scenes his face looked like my son's and slowly morphed into his own.

I woke up from the dream drenched in sweat. I sat straight up in my bed and said thank you God for being who you are and your faithfulness. I knew that God had answered my prayers regarding helping me to forgive my mother's friend and what he did to me. I clearly understood exactly what message God was conveying to me through that dream. I even understood why in the dream his face morphed into my son's and vice versa. We do not know what others have been through in their lives to cause them to do the things that they do. As believers we are required to forgive those that trespass against us and not seek vengeance, for vengeance belongs to the Lord (Romans 12:19 "Do not take revenge, my dear friends, but leave room for God's wrath, for it is written: It is mine to avenge; I will repay, says the Lord").

Forgiveness and not seeking vengeance does not mean that we condone what the person said or did. It also does not mean we have to keep in contact or maintain a relationship with the person or people who hurt us. Forgiveness is necessary for our healing, peace, spirituality and to receive God's favor more abundantly by remaining faithful and adhering to His word. Forgiveness also gives us the power to let go, move on and stop being held captive mentally and emotionally by what happened to us. It is necessary for us to forgive others for what they have done to us, in order for God to forgive us for what we have done to and against Him and others. We have all sinned and fall short of the glory of God. (Colossians 3:13-15 "Bear with each other and forgive one another if any of you has a grievance against someone. Forgive as the Lord forgave you. And over all these virtues put on love, which binds them all together in perfect unity. Let the peace of Christ rule in your hearts, since as members of one body, you were called to peace. And be thankful").

CHAPTER

8

❧

MENTAL HEALTH ISSUES

I PREVIOUSLY MENTIONED THAT MY GRANDMOTHER, MOTHER AND SOME other relatives battled mental health issues and suffered from alcohol use disorder. My grandmother was not officially diagnosed with a mental health issue until she was in her 70's but displayed symptoms for decades prior to her diagnosis. Due to her also engaging in alcohol use when she displayed symptoms of her mental health issue, we assumed it was due to her being under the influence of alcohol and did not realize she was battling a mental health issue. What we later learned after her diagnosis is that she was probably using alcohol to self-medicate to cope with the symptoms of her mental health issue.

My mother received a diagnosis of depression when she was in her late 30's. But since she was not medication compliant and still displaying symptoms of her depression, she also used alcohol to cope with her symptoms. Using alcohol, substances and other vices are very common coping mechanisms for individuals who suffer from mental health issues.

I noticed as a teenager that I periodically experienced drastic fluctuations in my mood. Some days, I would wake up feeling like I was on top of the world and other days I could barely pull myself out of bed because I was so depressed. At that age, I did not have a clear understanding of mental health or even what it meant when my mother said that she was diagnosed with depression and was prescribed medication. I assumed my drastic mood fluctuations were a direct result of being bullied at school and having a challenging home life. Honestly, I am not sure I would have been able to fully comprehend that I suffered from Bipolar Affective Disorder at that age.

Bipolar Affective Disorder, formerly known as Depression, is a neurobiological brain disorder that affects over 2 million Americans. Bipolar Disorder causes radical shifts in moods, energy and the ability to carry out everyday tasks. Individuals with Bipolar Disorder experience periods of intense emotions and changes in behavior called "mood episodes" for days for even weeks at a time. Depressive moods can cause a person to feel a strong sense of sadness with low energy and motivation. Manic episodes are the opposite of depressive episodes. Individuals can feel energetic, optimistic and in some occasions even euphoric which can lead to irrational and impulsive decision making. The type and intensity of Bipolar Disorder can vary from person to person. I was recently diagnosed and prescribed medication to help manage the symptoms associated with Bipolar Affective Disorder, but not before going down the "rabbit hole" of trying to self-medicate with food and alcohol to soothe and help cope with the symptoms.

I was introduced to alcohol on my 16th birthday. Prior to that day I had tried to innocently take a sip every now and then of my mother's drink when she wasn't looking, but the taste was so vile to me that I would immediately spit it out. My mother and one of her girlfriends were at our apartment, talking, laughing, listening to music and having a few drinks. My mother told me that I had my usual duties of playing the DJ and refilling drinks. She instructed me to grab her and her girlfriend another drink out of the refrigerator. My mother's friend asked her if she had anything a little stronger than what they had been drinking. My mother replied, "I have some whiskey. You want some of that?" My mother's friend nodded her head yes and said "and make it a double." My mother laughed and said "Girl it's Chelle's birthday, not yours." My mother's friend started laughing too, "Well tell Chelle to make herself one too. One drink won't hurt her."

My mother hesitated for a moment before telling me to make us all a drink. "But you are only getting this one drink because it's your birthday. You are almost grown and I am sure you have been sneaking and drinking with your little fast friends anyway." She was wrong. I hated the taste of alcohol when I had previously snuck a taste of her drink. However, I was willing to try it this one time. How bad could it be? My mother and her friends seemed to enjoy it on occasion. It must not be too bad. It made me feel "mature" having a drink with my mom and her friend. It made me feel like I was one of the girls for once.

When I took the first sip of the whiskey and Pepsi-Cola concoction, I was sure that I was going to immediately vomit. My face was beyond contorted and I stuck my tongue out of my mouth because it was on fire "Yuck that was disgusting. I don't want any more of that." My mom snapped back "Girl you better not waste that drink. Finish that glass. You shouldn't have asked for it." I didn't ask for it, I thought to myself. I knew there was no winning a debate with my mom so I gulped it down.

My throat was burning and I initially felt extremely nauseous, so I went to lie down in my bed. After a few minutes of lying there, I did not feel sick anymore. I actually felt pretty good and very relaxed. The music my mother was playing sounded exceptionally good and I had the urge to get up and dance. My usual down in the dumps, woe is me, demeanor had disappeared. At that moment, I felt like I had discovered a magic potion to cure all of my problems. I could not remember when I had felt as upbeat, free and courageous. (I would discover the error in my thinking later in life.)

I was feeling so good that I asked my mom if I could pour myself another drink and to my surprise, she told me that I could have one more. I couldn't believe that I was now part of the fun, laughter, yelling and dancing that I only witnessed and overheard from behind the curtain that separated my sleeping area from the living room. I am not sure how long we were up talking, laughing and dancing that night. What I do know is that when I woke up the next morning, my head felt like someone had hit me in the head with a brick multiple times. My mouth was dry, my body ached and I felt sicker to my stomach than I had ever felt before.

I knew that I felt this way because I had consumed alcohol but this felt worse than the flu. For some reason I knew that this feeling would not prevent me from drinking alcohol again because even though I got sick, it made me feel better temporarily. I told myself that I just drank the "wrong kind" of alcohol. The next time I drank alcohol I would remember to drink wine; something with less alcohol content. I would later learn that the problem was not the kind of alcohol I drank that day. The problem was I had something much deeper going on that no amount or kind of alcohol could cure.

Despite the fact that I felt extremely ill after my first encounter with alcohol, I drank alcohol a few more times over the next several years. At first, it was very seldom because I was a new mom and working full time. I would only drink wine or fruity drinks because I did not like the taste of alcohol and that was usually on a special occasion. As time went on and life started to happen, my alcohol consumption slowly started to increase. As I found myself feeling depressed more often I found myself craving alcohol more often to cope.

I rarely drank during the weekdays, but was beginning to engage in alcohol at least one day of most weekends. I convinced myself that because I worked all week, kept a clean home, was a loving and caring mother to my children, volunteered in the community and attended church that I deserved a little "treat" on the weekend to relax and unwind from the hustle and bustle of the workweek. The Bible even referenced drinking wine (I am aware that my theory and rationalization for drinking alcohol took those scriptures out of context). It helped me to cope with my anxiety, depression, and sleep issues (at least I thought it did until I became more educated about the negative effects of alcohol and realized that it made all those symptoms worse). I eventually learned the hard way that indulging in alcohol and using it to self-medicate was not the solution to my issues.

Since I was only consuming alcohol on the weekends and I was still handling my responsibilities, I did not believe that my drinking was an issue. I usually just drank wine at home while cleaning or watching movies. In my opinion the alcohol just helped to balance out my mood. I did not feel as anxious or depressed when I was drinking. I even felt more confident and outspoken. This was a feeling that I never experienced without alcohol in my childhood or adult years.

On occasion a loved one or friend would mention that I was more argumentative and had a quick temper when I consumed alcohol but in my opinion they were just saying that because I actually spoke my mind and stood up for myself when I was drinking alcohol and they had gotten used to the docile; push over version of me. I did notice that I was more courageous and not afraid to speak my mind when I consumed alcohol. I would not let people get away with the usual snide comments or statements.

I can recall an incident when a friend of mine and I were at my home. Our kids were at a sleepover and we were watching movies and drinking some wine. We were talking about old times, relationships, family and kids. We were having a good time at first. However, she brought up a past event and made a statement about a mutual friend that I did not agree with. I was shocked that she would say something like that about our friend. I told her that I did not agree with her and asked her not to speak ill of this friend in my presence. She went on to say that she was an adult and would say whatever she liked. I told her that if she chose to continue to talk about our friend in that manner that I would have to ask her to leave my home. I could immediately see the look of hurt on her face. She was shocked that I would suggest that she leave my home because of that reason. After saying a few more choice words to me, she put on her coat and left. Our friendship was never quite the same after that evening. I had to wonder if we were not engaging in alcohol would I have actually suggested that she leave even though I did not like the fact that she was talking about a mutual friend. I believe had we not been drinking, I would have thought of a clever way to redirect the conversation instead of giving that ultimatum. I began to see the negative impact that alcohol could have on people and relationships.

I recognized that I had developed an unhealthy relationship with alcohol but I wasn't sure what to do about it. I had started to use alcohol to deal with situations and emotions that I should have been praying to God about instead. It seemed like most of my social circle consumed alcohol and when I did try to abstain from it completely I felt extremely uncomfortable especially in social settings. I knew plenty of people who drank alcohol, but I didn't know a single person who was successfully practicing abstinence after they had an unhealthy relationship with alcohol. I felt exceptionally anxious when I refrained from drinking alcohol for extended periods of time and would eventually begin overeating to soothe the anxiety symptoms and fill that sugar craving due to the absence of alcohol.

I was able to navigate the workweek easily without thinking about or drinking alcohol, but I looked forward to the weekend when I could relax and have a few drinks. It was difficult to talk to anyone about my alcohol use because there is such a stigma associated with people, especially women who indulge in alcohol. I was a Christian, mother, wife, college educated, professional woman, who was active in the community but secretly struggled with using alcohol to cope with anxiety and depression symptoms. I was ashamed to discuss it or ask anyone close to me for advice or help. I searched online for support groups in my area and began to attend virtual and in-person support meetings.

I soon realized that I was not alone. There were many professional Christian women who also struggled with their mental health and had developed an unhealthy relationship with alcohol. The meetings were helpful and I was able to drastically reduce my alcohol intake; only rarely engaging in alcohol use. But, it wasn't until I heard an unforgettable sermon and experienced a life altering event that I was able to achieve complete abstinence from alcohol.

I moved away from the small town that I grew up in several years ago. My daughters still reside there so I visit often. On this particular weekend I was in town for a housewarming party. Whenever I am in town on a Sunday I try to make sure that I visit my former church home. I love my pastor and first lady at my new church. But visiting my former church is always an awesome experience and feels like home.

My former pastor's sermon topic was titled "Almost." In his sermon he discussed that almost being saved wasn't good enough to get you into heaven. He asked the congregation how they would feel or what they would do if at the end of this life they were told that they almost made it to heaven but it was just one thing that prevented them from being saved and having eternal life. He encouraged the congregation to take an assessment of their life and determine if there was something that could or would prevent them from being saved and going to heaven.

I immediately knew that my one thing was alcohol. Although I wasn't drinking on a regular basis at that time, I knew that I still had an unhealthy relationship with it because I still thought about drinking when I was trying to cope with stress, anxiety or depression. I also believed that engaging in alcohol use even just occasionally was keeping me from fully operating in my gift and fulfilling His purpose for me. On occasion, I was still turning to alcohol to deal with issues that I should have been praying about and asking for God's help with. I am not saying that is the case for everyone, but I believe alcohol was becoming a hindrance and impacting my relationship with God and others.

After hearing that sermon, I began to pray to God to reveal and remove anything from me that was not of His will. I asked him to help me to break any unhealthy habits or behaviors that remained in my life, so that I could clearly identify and operate in my gift in order to fulfill the purpose that He has for my life. 17 days later, He answered my prayers in a way that I could not have imagined in my wildest dreams and I have some pretty wild ones.

"Good Morning Michelle. How are you feeling today." a nurse asked me. "I am feeling fine. Where am I?" I replied, while lying on my back in a very small bed looking around a room that definitely was not in my own home. I could tell by the decor of the room and sounds of the medical equipment coming from the hallway that I was in some kind of health care or medical facility. What I didn't know immediately was how I had gotten there. While I was trying to piece my memories together in an attempt to figure out what was going on, the nurse interrupted my thoughts by asking me the very thing that I was pondering over "Do you remember how you got here Michelle?" I shook my head "No, I don't."

As I tried to get up from the bed, the nurse instructed me to take it easy and said "You are at a Behavioral Health Center and you are safe. Your family brought you into the emergency room on Wednesday evening because they were concerned about some of the statements that you were making about wanting to see your deceased mother and the fact that you seemed to be in a semi-conscious state of mind." My head was spinning at this point. "Wednesday?" I asked in disbelief. "What day is today?" I questioned. "Today is Friday," she said. My mind and thoughts were so foggy. I could remember bits and pieces of images but I was unable to decipher if they had been a dream or reality.

She went on to say that my family had advised her that I had not slept in several days prior to the episode that happened on Wednesday that prompted them to bring me into the emergency room. This was a lot to take in. If I was still drinking alcohol I would have thought that I may have been consuming alcohol prior to this incident and that was the cause for my foggy memories. But I knew I had not drank alcohol in quite a while so that could not be the cause. I had no idea what could have prompted this episode to happen to me. I had never had anything like this happen to me before.

When I called my husband he was able to provide me with more details and jog my memory a little. He reminded me that I had been working on writing my book and working long hours. He said that I had not gotten more than four or five hours of sleep total in the four days prior to this episode. He began to remind me of some of the things I had said to him. When he mentioned some of the things that I had said I did vaguely remember them, but I thought I was dreaming and the entire time I was "awake". He said that I told him that I wanted to see my mother who is deceased. I asked him if I seemed like I was trying to commit suicide. He assured me that was not the case. He said that I was behaving like I actually saw her or had just seen her (She passed away 8 years ago). I was calling out for our daughters who live in another state. I was reaching out for our son who lives in the same town but was at work at the time. He said that I asked him if he promised not to let anyone hurt me because I wasn't feeling like myself. He emphasized that he understood everything I was asking and the questions made sense, but he could tell that I was not in a fully conscious state of mind and something was wrong. He said that he and my daughters tried to delay taking me to the hospital. They tried to let me get some sleep to identify if sleep deprivation was causing the episode. But because I kept trying to get up and walk around, they were afraid that I may fall and hurt myself and wanted to ensure that I was safe. He told me that the two things that I kept repeating while I was in that state of mind were "Heaven is real, babe" and "Take me to the family reunion to see my family."

I am not sure if he could tell by the sound of my voice that I was crying but tears were streaming down my face. Everything that he was saying to me coincided with what I now remembered seeing, but thought I was dreaming. During this "dream" I saw, heard and felt my deceased mother's presence from a distance. She was happy and well; not sick and frail like when she passed away. I dreamed (or had what I thought was a dream) that I was at a family reunion and saw all of my family members there having a wonderful time, even the ones who had passed on. Everyone was young and healthy. They looked so much happier and more peaceful than when they had passed away.

I saw a place that I knew had to be in heaven because it was more beautiful than any place on earth that I had ever seen. The colors were so vivid and bright. I also saw the most massive and exquisite sanctuary imaginable. This sanctuary looked more like a magnificent stadium cathedral. It had to seat hundreds of thousands of people and it was filled to capacity. The choir was colossal and they were singing and playing the most beautiful music that I had ever heard. It brought tears to my eyes just hearing it.

I heard my husband's voice on the other end of the phone saying "Hello, Hello?" I had been daydreaming again. He shared that there was something else he needed to tell me. My husband reluctantly broke the news to me that I had been diagnosed with Bipolar Affective Disorder and had experienced a hypomanic episode triggered by increased stress and lack of sleep. He explained that I had been prescribed some medication and the doctor suggested that I stay at the behavioral health center for a couple of more days so they could observe how I responded to it. Although my family was extremely supportive throughout this ordeal, I had never felt more scared, lonely and vulnerable. But, I also found comfort in finally knowing why my moods always fluctuated so drastically and having a treatment plan to follow.

I know that God used this episode to help me identify this underlying issue so that I could get help and stop reverting to alcohol to try and cope with the symptoms of my illness. I was almost halfway through writing this book prior to this episode happening. I initially planned to discuss my faith and what God had done in my life, but the primary focus of the original book was going to be about the fasting and weight loss element in the program. However, during the episode I experienced, I also saw myself writing a book. I literally saw my hand writing the manuscript and suddenly while I was sitting at my desk writing a pencil started to erase all of the letter I's from the pages of the manuscript that I had written. Seeing that image in conjunction with everything else that was revealed to me during this "episode" I knew that I needed to start this book over from the beginning to ensure that the focus was on Him, His grace, His mercy and His healing power. I needed to remove myself from the equation because I did not and could not do anything without him. (Jeremiah 29:11-13 "For I know the plans I have for you, declares the Lord, plans to prosper you and not to harm you, plans to give you hope and a future. Then you will call on me and come and pray to me and I will listen to you. You will seek me and find me when you seek me with all your heart").

CHAPTER
9

✾

PARENTAL GUILT

I BELIEVE THAT IF MOST PARENTS ARE HONEST, THEY HAVE FELT SOME form of parental guilt. A more common term is "Mommy Guilt." But with so many different family dynamics and structures in our society, I wanted to be inclusive and refer to it as parental guilt. I had my first daughter at the age of 17 and knew very little about parenthood aside from what I read in all of the popular parenting books and magazines. I knew that I wanted to break the cycle of how I was raised and generational issues with my children but honestly did not know exactly how to achieve that.

I was operating in a state of uncertainty from the time she was an infant through her teenage years. I felt the most parental guilt with my oldest daughter because of my age and she was my first child. I felt a little more experienced raising my younger daughter and son. But my oldest daughter is definitely responsible for a few of my gray hairs. I was confused and concerned about which foods to feed her, what content she was exposed to, schools she attended, extracurricular activities she was involved in, her friends, dating choices and discipline. The list goes on and on.

Structure and discipline were probably two of the things that I struggled with the most, especially after going through a divorce.

I internally battled with being too strict or not being strict enough. I grappled even more with the possible consequences of making the wrong choice. I wanted my children to enjoy their youth but also wanted to ensure that I was raising them to be God-fearing, responsible and productive individuals. Parenthood is one of those things that is so important and you don't get a second chance if and when you mess up. Making mistakes and "messing up" does not constitute being a bad parent. It just makes us human. There is no instruction manual that comes along with raising children.

I can recall having a conversation with my oldest daughter about her childhood. We were discussing her memories of it. I felt so guilty about so many things ranging from being a young mom to not being able to provide her with all of the material things that I thought that she wanted and needed. Due to growing up poor, I was afraid and concerned of returning to poverty and always tried to make sure I had a decent paying job so I could provide for my children. I never wanted them to go without or get teased and bullied in school the way that I did because of how they dressed or what they did not have. I wanted to make sure they had nice clothes and shoes. I wanted to make sure that I could afford to send them on all of the school trips and they could participate in any clubs or activities that they chose. However, my daughter did not mention any of that. She mentioned that she just wished I didn't have to work so much and could have stayed home with her more.

I was a little shocked. I wished I could have stayed home with her more also, but I thought she would have mentioned something about the things that I couldn't provide for her or about me being so young and inexperienced. She just wanted to spend more time with me. I had been concerned and worried about all of the wrong things. Due to my childhood, I automatically thought I was doing the right thing by working hard to provide for her but I missed the mark. She wanted me to be at home with her and felt I had missed some significant events in her youth. I was devastated and heartbroken. I felt so bad that I worked so much and wasn't able to be at home with her more and attend those events.

My parental guilt did not end with my oldest daughter though.

When my other children dated someone who did not have their best interest at heart and they experienced heartbreak, I also felt parental guilt. I felt guilty because I had not set the best example for them. I had not provided them the tools they needed to screen a potential partner to identify if they were suitable to date and engage in a relationship with. My relationship with their father had ended in divorce. Like my mother was unable to give me the level of compassion and empathy that I required, I did not set the greatest example of how to select a partner to date or have a relationship with. I prepared them for life in many other ways but I may have failed them in that area.

I also felt tremendous guilt when I occasionally saw them engage in any type of alcohol use. None of my children have an unhealthy relationship with alcohol, but I have on occasion heard them say that they were stressed or upset and then have a couple of glasses of wine. Of course, this is a red flag for me because of our family history and I know that my unhealthy relationship with alcohol started with me trying to soothe my wounds and manage my emotions and mood.

I experience a feeling of guilt associated with this because I wonder if they have learned to associate emotions with alcohol use from me. I never want to be the reason or cause that any of my children stumble in their lives. My sole mission as a mother was to give them the best lives possible by breaking unhealthy generational patterns and giving them the tools to use in life that I did not have. But I am not perfect and I failed in some areas. I learned a lot along this journey called parenthood and I am a better Christian, wife, mother, grandmother and bonus mom because of it. There were a lot of ups and downs; bumps and bruises but it resulted in tremendous overall growth as a parent. God covered my children and I through it all. (Psalm 55:22 "Cast your cares on the Lord and he will sustain you. He will never let the righteous be shaken"). (Proverbs 14:26 "Whoever fears the Lord has a secure fortress and for their children it will be a refuge").

CHAPTER
10

✦

ACCEPTANCE & THE UNCONDITIONAL LOVE OF GOD

PSYCHOLOGICAL ACCEPTANCE CAN BE DEFINED AS THE ACTIVE EMBRACING of subjective experiences, particularly distressing experiences. In general and everyday life acceptance can be defined as the action or process of being received as adequate or suitable, often related to being admitted into a group. I needed to embrace psychological acceptance to deal with the trauma and abuse that I experienced throughout my life. I struggled with lacking general acceptance into groups of friends and schoolmates as a child. I also had an extremely difficult time tolerating and accepting the behavior of those who did not display acceptance and the unconditional love of God to others; especially from other believers. (I eventually recognized the error in my way of thinking and realized that if I was judging them because of how they behaved, I wasn't displaying the unconditional love of God either). Because I longed for acceptance throughout my adolescent years and I knew first-hand how being an outcast or lacking acceptance from others can negatively impact an individual's life and self-image, I was extremely intolerant of anyone who displayed a lack of respect, empathy, and acceptance of other people due to their differences or challenges.

Surprisingly enough I witnessed and experienced a lack of unconditional love, empathy, and acceptance in the church, the one place that everyone should be accepted and welcome. Some newcomers and visitors did not always receive a warm welcome and were sometimes treated in a dismissive manner by long standing members. They would treat these visitors as if attending church was a request for membership to an exclusive club where everyone had to meet a specific criteria in order to gain access instead of the all-inclusive house of God where everyone should be welcome to come pray, worship, learn more about God and His word and to fellowship with other believers that church is supposed to be.

This was gut-wrenching to me because the church is where people often come when they are struggling mentally, physically, emotionally and spiritually. They may be feeling hopeless; even suicidal and have absolutely nowhere else to turn and managed to make it into the house of God to only be greeted with eye rolls, dirty looks and crass comments. I mentioned earlier in this book about how we can take it upon ourselves to add a value system to what we believe is a sin and treat people unfairly due to circumstances that may be beyond their control. I have seen members of the LGBTQIA+ community (which includes but not limited to lesbian, gay, bisexual, transgender, intersex, and asexual individuals), people who were homeless, have been arrested, had an abortion, suffer from mental health issues, intellectual disabilities, alcohol, and substance use disorders treated poorly and rejected because of their current situation, differences, and challenges. I never understood why this type of behavior was prevalent in the church when treating anyone this way was judgmental and was not in alignment with God's word.

I make an effort to try and be kind and friendly to everyone regardless of their situation because I understand that anyone can be just a missed paycheck away from facing homelessness, one bad decision away from being arrested or being a convicted felon, or one situation away from being diagnosed with having a mental health or psychological disorder. I often wondered to myself when I witnessed these types of interactions, how did we as believers expect to convince people to accept Christ who we cannot see as their Lord and savior and we were unable to accept, help, and welcome those in need who we see and interact with daily?

I can recall participating in a church outreach event to provide food and supplies such as personal care items, socks and gloves to the homeless. I was so eager to be a part of an effort that fulfilled a desperate need in our community. We arrived at the destination and began to pass out the food items and supplies. The people who received the supplies were extremely grateful. Some of them wanted to engage in lengthy conversations or even hug myself and the others who gave them the much needed items. This warmed my heart, because I recalled the days when I had slept in the back of my mother's friend's truck camper, and it was not a pleasant experience. I realized that a sudden unfortunate situation could cause me to lose my job and I would be in the same position that they were currently. I was honored to talk to, pray with or give them a hug because I was helping God's people who were in need.

After I hugged one of the gentlemen who was ecstatic to receive the items we were passing out, one of the church members handed me some hand sanitizer and leaned in and whispered "Be careful about touching them. Many of them are sick and have diseases." Because of my experience with being temporarily homeless, I was immediately offended and appalled. I realized that technically, she was probably correct about some of the people we were helping having diseases because unfortunately due to their living conditions they did not have access to running water, soap, sanitizer and other items needed to maintain proper hygiene. But I couldn't help myself from becoming upset by the timing and nature of the statement. I thought to myself that many people who are not homeless are sick and have diseases that we could possibly contract. Pre-Covid, I did not go around sanitizing my hands every time I gave someone a hug.

At my former church, there was actually a hugging ministry where there was a time designated during church service for members to walk around the sanctuary to greet and hug everyone. It was heartbreaking that in addition to those individuals having to endure living in substandard conditions that they also were being prejudged and discriminated against by the church members who were supposed to be there to offer aid and assistance. I wholeheartedly believe that the God I serve will provide a layer of protection around me especially when I am doing His will. So in the midst of doing so, contracting an illness or disease has never crossed my mind. My favorite scripture is Matthew 25:40 because it keeps and reminds me to be humble, loving and kind to everyone despite their past, circumstances, struggles or current situation and reminds me that how I treat others who are also God's children is also how I am treating God. ("The King will reply, Truly I tell you, whatever you did for one of the least of these brothers and sisters of mine, you did for me").

In addition to my personal experience with being treated like an outcast and not being accepted throughout periods of my life, I also had family members and loved ones who dealt with personal struggles and challenges that caused them to be ostracized. It was agonizing when a close relative who was diagnosed as being mildly mentally disabled experienced this type of treatment. It is heartbreaking enough when people mistreat adults, but it is nearly unbearable when children are treated in a manner that disregards their feelings. Medical professionals who are expected to have a higher level of education, subject matter knowledge and protocol have referred to his condition inaccurately in his presence and used a derogatory term that should no longer be used to describe his disability.

When he was about five or six years old, a woman standing in line behind me at the grocery store overheard me talking to him and asked me if he could talk as if he wasn't standing right beside me and couldn't hear her . He was delayed with learning to speak and was responding to me with a limited vocabulary of words. But I could not understand for the life of me what would possess someone or give them the audacity to ask a complete stranger such a personal question especially in the presence of the child they are inquiring about. Other strangers have approached us and blatantly asked "What's wrong with him?" I must admit that I have responded to them from my flesh at times, because it is so challenging to control your emotions and keep your composure when someone disrespects someone that you love, especially a defenseless child. As I matured in my faith, I learned to pray for them, take the opportunity to educate them and combat their negativity with the word of God.

Many years ago an associate of mine disclosed to me that she had an abortion. She was in a violent domestic relationship, already had two children, one of which was only four months old at the time and had just found out she was pregnant again. She was living in a housing project in a high crime area and was unemployed at the time because she had just had her youngest child. She confided that her boyfriend had abused her a few days prior to our conversation, and I could see that her eye was still badly bruised.

She was holding their baby when he hit her the first time. In an effort to ensure that he did not accidently hit the baby she laid the baby down on the couch. Her boyfriend continued to hit, punch her and pull her hair. During the altercation, the infant rolled off of the couch. Thankfully, the baby was not injured, but my friend knew that she could not remain in that relationship but she had nowhere else to go. She was also afraid that the baby she was carrying may have been seriously injured and could possibly be born with complications or disabilities due to the severity of the attack while she was still in the early stages of her pregnancy.

She felt an extreme amount of guilt because the abusive relationship she was in was now beginning to affect her children. She was only 18 years old at the time and originally moved in with her boyfriend to escape an abusive home life, so she did not have a support system. She had no idea how she would care for her other two children. When she sought advice, prayer and help from her church family, she was told that abortion was a sin and she would burn in hell if she followed through with it.

She began to cry uncontrollably after repeating this to me. I prayed for her and told her that I did not believe that the God we served operated in that manner. Our God knows all things, sees all things and can heal all things. I gave her the name of a local women's shelter that could help her find housing, employment and childcare. I also reminded her that God knows our hearts and He solely has the final say, not the church (Micah 7:19 "You will again have compassion on us; you will tread our sins underfoot and hurl all our iniquities into the depths of the sea").

Many individuals who are part of the LGBTQIA+ community have also been repudiated by their church, discriminated against in their workplace and community and even physically and sexually assaulted. One of my clients suffered from a condition called "Gynecomastia" which caused him to have enlarged breast tissue caused by a hormonal imbalance. His breast tissue was enlarged because his body produced more estrogen than normal for a male. Estrogen and testosterone are considered as the two main female and male sex hormones, so this hormone imbalance also impacted his sexual functionality. He had to deal with people close to him spreading rumors that the reason he had breasts and had a feminine voice was because he was taking hormone pills to appear more feminine. When in fact he was taking hormone pills to increase his testosterone levels in an effort to balance his hormones and appear less feminine.

He was often called derogatory names due to his femininity and sexual preference and was physically assaulted on multiple occasions. As a teenager, he experienced being sexually assaulted by multiple men who told him that since he wanted to act like a girl they were going to treat him like one. He loved God, went to church and asked members of his church to pray for him to be healed. He was told that his sexuality was a choice and that he was choosing to sin against God. Church members told him that there is no such thing as being born homosexual and he should just stop being attracted to men. We just never know what people are dealing with when we encounter them and I believe that is why God's word instructs us to love and treat others how we want to be loved and treated (Mark 12:30-31 "Love the Lord your God with all your heart, with all your soul and with all your mind and with all your strength. The second is this: Love your neighbor as yourself. There is no commandment greater than these").

I struggled with demonstrating unconditional love, acceptance and forgiveness of people, especially believers who discriminate against the LGBTQIA+ or any other minority group of individuals because their life is challenging enough without the extra drama or hatred. I loathed when spiritual leaders used the Bible to perpetuate discrimination or lack of acceptance for specific groups of people. I have heard believers say things like they cannot wear or display the rainbow anymore because it is a symbol that is now associated with the LGBTQIA+ community and their "lifestyle" is a sin against God. Comments like these always shock me for two reasons (1) one I absolutely love rainbows and (2) I can't understand how a believer in God says that they are unable to wear or display a rainbow which signifies a covenant between God and all living creatures on earth which certainly includes the LGBTQIA+ community and all other minority groups of individuals. (Genesis 9:16 "Whenever the rainbow appears in the clouds, I will see it and remember the everlasting covenant between God and all living creatures of every kind on the earth"). There are so many things that as mere humans we just do not understand and are unable to comprehend. I truly believe that is why the Bible emphasizes the importance of being empathetic, compassionate, non-judgmental of others, nor leaning on our own understanding. (I Peter 3:8 "Finally all of you, be like-minded, be sympathetic, love one another, be compassionate and humble"). As my current pastor always says, "We have to ensure that we are viewing the world through our spiritual eyeglasses and not looking at and navigating it through the world's view."

When I first accepted Jesus Christ as my personal Lord and savior, began to learn more about God, His word and attended church every Sunday, I was so inspired, motivated and on fire for God. I was so excited to be in the house of the Lord and take my life in the right direction. I could not wait to share my gifts and help more in the community. At the time, I was a recently divorced mother of three teenagers. I was glad to find a church home and positive activities that my children and I could participate in. Each week as I listened to the pastor speak, I eagerly awaited to identify how my kids and I could be used by God in a ministry. The pastor often spoke about not having enough help from the members of the church. He said that it seemed like the same five or 10 people were doing all of the work in the church and that was unfair because we had hundreds of members.

One Sunday, he mentioned that the church was in need of an usher and some additional people to help clean the church on Saturday mornings. I thought to myself, my kids and I could definitely do that. The pastor always advised new members to just let him know if there was a ministry that we were interested in. I told him that I would be interested in serving as an usher and that my kids and I could help clean the church on Saturdays. He was appreciative and thrilled stating that we could start the upcoming Saturday.

When my kids and I arrived the following Saturday, I instructed my son to start collecting the trash from the classrooms, bathrooms and kitchen area. I told my daughters that one of them could pick up the chairs and items off of the floor and the other one could start vacuuming the floors. I let them know that I was going to start cleaning the restrooms. It felt rewarding to be volunteering our time to tidy up God's house. Not long after I started cleaning the main restroom, I heard some commotion coming from one of the classrooms. I immediately recognized my son's voice, but I couldn't identify who the woman was that sounded as if she was chastising him about something. When I entered the classroom, the woman immediately asked me if I was his mother and did I know he was playing around in one of the classrooms.

My son tried to interject, but I hushed him and tried to explain to the woman what we were doing there and that we had cleared it with the pastor. She was very short and rude with me and told me if I was going to bring all of my kids there on the weekends that I needed to watch them and that my son who was a teenager at the time could not be left unattended in the classrooms. My kids were frustrated with how the woman spoke to us when we were trying to help out and do a good deed.

The following Sunday was also my first day as an usher. Despite the fact that we had an unpleasant experience the previous day, I was still excited and a little nervous about my first day serving as an usher. I was there on time and trying to remember everything that I needed to do. The person who had trained me was really nice and patient with me, but she was not going to be there on my first day and I would be ushering with someone else. The music began and some members started proceeding into the sanctuary. I was greeting everyone as they walked in and handing out programs for the service.

I felt someone firmly grab my arm and pull me backwards out of the sanctuary doors and into the church foyer. I turned around and saw it was another one of the ushers. She held onto my arm and led me into a classroom in the back of the building and shut the door behind us. The way that she grabbed my arm and held on to it, I knew that something serious must be going on. I was praying that there was nothing wrong with my kids who were in another area of the church. The usher pushed me against the wall with an irritated expression on her face and asked "Do you have a slip on?" "Excuse me?" I asked to ensure that I heard her correctly. "Yes, a slip? You do know what a slip is, don't you?"

I could not believe my ears. I could not believe that she had dragged me out of the sanctuary and brought me back here to ask me about a slip. I tried to hold my composure and respond respectfully because she was my elder. "Yes I know what a slip is but I did not realize that I was required to wear one since I have on a thick black cotton knee length skirt. I also do not own a slip." "Well, I suggest that you purchase one if you want to remain on the Usher Board and serve as an usher. This is the house of the Lord and you should have on proper attire when you are in His house." I was flabbergasted. The only respectful response that I could conjure up was "Yes, ma'am." My mother raised us to have a great respect for the house of the Lord and to dress appropriately. There was nothing inappropriate about the clothing I was wearing. I felt that usher wanted to display and exercise her authority in that ministry.

That incident definitely robbed me of some of the joy and excitement that I originally had about serving on different ministries in the church. I was starting to realize why some of the members may not be active in ministries if they were treated in the manner that I was. However, I had a love and respect for the pastor and first lady and was determined not to let a few people or isolated incidents deter my efforts.

My kids and I attended a Christmas party at the church a few months later. The kids had taken off to talk to some friends as I walked around the fellowship hall speaking to everyone. After I finished making my rounds, I went over to the refreshment table to get some chips and a soda. One of the members that I barely knew approached me. I smiled and said hello. She spoke and said that she was surprised to see me there since I hadn't attended many of the previous events at the church. I told her that yes I was trying to make sure to come to more church events so that I could mingle and meet other church members. Then she asked me with a straight face "Are you sure that you didn't just come to the Christmas Party for the free food and gifts for the kids?" She gave a little chuckle and walked off.

I did not know her well enough to know what to make of her comments. I was still significantly overweight at the time and wasn't sure if she was taking a jab at me about my weight or not. Since there were some other people standing nearby, I prayed that they did not hear her comment. I didn't even eat the chips and soda that I had put on a plate. Her comment, especially at an event that was being held in the church and supposed to be a celebration of the birth of Christ spoiled my appetite. If my kids had not been having such a good time, I would have immediately left.

I have witnessed several situations like this in various churches and it is sad, but I refuse to let a few unpleasant experiences ruin the joy I experience when I am in the house of the Lord. I had to remember that regardless of how others may behave, they were still my brothers and sisters in Christ and I had to exercise tolerance, patience, and acceptance. I had to remember that I was working and coming to church for Him not for them (Matthew 5:44 But I tell you, love your enemies and pray for those who persecute you.)

I have shared my truth and cleaned out the debris that lingered inside of me from my life experiences. These bad experiences hindered me from becoming the best version of me. With God's help I purified my heart. I was able to forgive and ask for forgiveness with a clean heart. I can now move on to Phase III of this process which is to change and rebuild my core.

PHASE

III

❁

CHANGE & REBUILD YOUR CORE

ITFELTGOODTOFREEMYSELFFROMTHEDEBRISTHATLINGEREDINSIDE of me from past experiences and shatter through the barriers aka glass ceiling that initially prevented me from becoming the best version of me. Now that I have cleared out all of the residue and negative feelings associated with it, I have the space and opportunity to begin changing and rebuilding my core. This phase is where I will put my best foot forward and decide what I want the best version of me to look like. I feel blessed, positive, free, and renewed and I want my personality, attitude and outer appearance to reflect that in every way. I want to have the love, peace and joy that I feel in my heart to radiate outward and prevent any external negative influences from penetrating inward. I must use a holistic approach that includes my mind, body and spirit to achieve this goal.

In order to have and maintain a positive mindset I must be extremely intentional about the things that I am exposed to, think about and meditate on. I have to be selective about the types of music, television, and social media that listen to, watch and engage in. In order to proactively promote a positive mindset I must start each day by praying, meditating, listening to, reading and watching material that promotes positive thinking and feelings. I must develop and maintain a gracious, humble and grateful spirit. It is imperative that I keep a daily journal where I will write down at least one thing that I can do to help or bless someone else each day and at least three different things that I am grateful for (I should not repeat anything on my gratitude list for at least 30 days).

It is crucial that I practice positive self-talk to build and maintain a positive self-image and to increase my self-esteem and feelings of self-worth. Even when I have an occasional negative thought or engage in negative self-talk, I must immediately identify the source and convert the negative self-talk or thoughts into positive self-talk and thoughts. It is essential that I conduct a daily assessment of my mood and emotions and make the necessary adjustments, such as when I experience the winter blues (or SAD-Seasonal Affective Disorder) I will listen to uplifting music, spend time with friends and family and/or use my light therapy lamp to improve my mood and reduce my symptoms.

Maintaining a positive network of friends and associates to interact with on a regular basis is vital. I need to be open to and actively seeking humor, laughter and having fun such as watching a comedy movie, playing cards or bowling with friends and family. Challenging myself to learn to swim and skate are also goals that I have set for myself. Engaging in these activities can organically reduce tension, improve mood (this is essential to my wellness because I am managing a mood disorder) and boost my immune system. In order to attain a high level of creativity, mental clarity and focus, I will practice healthy sleep habits (sleeping a minimum of 6-8 hours per evening and take a melatonin supplement if I am having difficulty falling or staying asleep), maintain a healthy and balanced diet, (intermittent fasting for a minimum of 18-20 hours per day and consuming plenty of water, lean protein, healthy fats, vegetables, fruits and other complex carbs) and follow an exercise regimen (30 to 60 consecutive minutes of exercise 5-6 days of the week that includes an alternating combination of cardio, resistance and strength training).

Exercise is also a mandatory part of my overall wellness because it causes my body to release the "neurochemicals of happiness" which are also known as Dopamine, Oxytocin, Serotonin and Endorphins. These chemicals can help to reduce stress, anxiety, depression and improve mood, sleep, and mental clarity. Last but not least, I will see my therapist on a regular basis to check in and ensure my mental health remains in a good place.

In addition to ensuring that I am promoting and maintaining positive mental health, I must also ensure that I am properly taking care of my body. I have already mentioned how I plan to eat a well-balanced diet, practice healthy sleep habits and follow an exercise regimen to care for the mental aspect of my holistic wellness plan which will also be beneficial for my body. Attire (stylish clothing), proper grooming (hair and nails), skin care (facials and saunas) and nurturing (massages and bubble baths) are also essential elements to properly care for my body. If I look good, I feel good. My appearance and how I care for myself is a key reflection of my self-love, self-image, self-esteem and self-worth. I realize that I will have challenging days and unexpected events happen that will prevent me from investing an exorbitant amount of time and effort into my physical appearance. But now that I have a holistic and balanced approach to managing my life those days should be few and far between.

I am an exclusive brand and the way I show up in the world every day is a reflection of my brand. I am also favored, divine, precious, elegant, unique and a direct reflection of God and that needs to be apparent daily. When I was struggling with depression and low self-esteem it was often obvious and reflective in my appearance. I put very little focus and effort into how I showed up in the world and self-care. I would often pull my hair back in a pony-tail or put on a baseball cap, put on an old baggy jogging suit and wore little or no make-up.

I also would not care about the types of food that I ate. My diet primarily consisted of junk food (candy, chips and cookies), highly processed food (from a box or can) and fast-food. During those dark periods, I rarely took the time to prepare a healthy balanced meal for myself such as broiled salmon and salad full of fresh vegetables, fruits, and nuts. I did not care how unhealthy the food was that I was putting in my body. I also did not follow an intermittent fasting lifestyle which I know is extremely healthy for my body.

Intermittent fasting helped me to lose over 70 pounds, reduced inflammation, overall body fat, reduced my blood pressure, lowered my risk of Type II diabetes (which my mother suffered with), reduced my bad cholesterol, increased mental clarity and brain fog. Intermittent fasting has also been proven to induce cellular repair through a process called autophagy. Autophagy involves the cells breaking down and metabolizing broken and dysfunctional proteins that build up in cells over time. Increased autophagy may provide protection against several diseases including cancer and neurodegenerative diseases such as Alzheimer's disease.

Going forward, I will ensure that I am living an intermittent fasting lifestyle and not constantly eating unhealthy foods throughout the day, which will give my body the opportunity to take a necessary break from continuously digesting food to naturally heal, restore and rejuvenate. I will eat to fuel my body with the essential nutrients needed to obtain optimal functionality and not out of boredom, for recreation or to cope with my feelings and emotions. I will eat high quality foods because my body is a temple and I will treat it as such. (I Corinthians 6:19-20 "Do you not know that your bodies are temples of the Holy Spirit, who is in you, whom you have received from God? You are not your own. You were bought at a price. Therefore honor God with your bodies").

Last but surely not least, I have to ensure that I am taking care of my spiritual health. This element is as equally crucial in becoming the best version of myself as the mind and body elements. I have to ensure that I am in daily communication with God and maintain a personal relationship with Him through reading and studying the Bible, (reading the daily devotional on Our Daily Bread app) prayer and constantly seeking his wisdom. When I am faced with challenges and struggles, I will refrain from submitting to my flesh and pursue resolutions by reading His word and allowing the Holy Spirit to direct and guide my path. I will attend weekly

Sunday school, church service and Bible study classes to increase my knowledge of Him and His word.

I will honor God with my time, talents and treasure by attending and supporting church outreach events, using my gift to help the ministry increase, collaborate and fellowship with other churches. I will faithfully tithe because it takes finances to maintain the church and provide resources for the community. (Matthew 6:21 "For where your treasure is, there your heart will be also"). I commit to carry myself in a manner which is in alignment with my Christian beliefs. I will engage in marketplace ministry in an appropriate manner and/or when a need or opportunity is identified. I will keep an open mind and be willing and ready to hear from God to be used as a vessel for His will and His way.

PHASE
IV

STRENGTHEN YOUR FAITH TO BECOME THE BEST VERSION OF YOU

Aftercompletingtheplanningandactionsneededtochange and rebuild my core, I need to focus on strengthening my faith to become the best version of me. In the previous phase, I worked on determining what the best version of me would look like. That consisted of the day to day surface level work that I need to do to ensure I will perform at my optimal level. I now get to decide what my future will also look like from a holistic perspective with all buckets full including mind, body and spirit. This is where I get to dream big and believe that my dreams will come true through manifestation. I just want to clarify that when I discuss manifestation, I am authentically speaking about it from a spiritual perspective. I am not alluding to the idea that all I have to do is think about something or put my dreams on a vision board and they will come true. I know exactly where my power comes from and that is solely from God.

However, I do support the idea that you receive the same energy back that you send out in the world. My belief is that if I faithfully operate within my gift that He has blessed me with, in addition to listening, trusting and obeying His word given to me to fulfill His purpose that He will open the floodgates and allow miraculous blessings to flow in my life, grant my dreams and the purest desires of my heart. Manifesting the life that I dream of will require me to increase my faith in what I pray and believe, which is that all things are possible through God who strengthens me and He makes no mistakes. I mention the fact that God does not make any mistakes because I have to reflect for just a moment on the trials and tribulations that he brought me through. In order to make a solid plan for my future I have to identify what lessons God needed me to learn from those extremely challenging situations so that I can be sure to use and apply those lessons learned and the knowledge gained through those experiences when and where it is deemed necessary. I know that no barrier that I shattered through or obstacle that I overcame was in vain. He had a purpose for each one.

I know that one of the lessons that he wanted me to learn was strength. Strength will be essential for the places and heights that God is trying to take me to. Another lesson that he was trying to teach me was to have faith and trust Him in all situations and not rely on my own understanding. I did not need to know the plan of how he was going to bring me out of the situation, I just needed to maintain faith in Him that He would bring me out. Using the fruits of the spirit; love, joy, peace, patience, kindness, goodness, faithfulness, gentleness and self-control to deal with challenging people and situations was another lesson that He needed me to learn. No matter what I do in this life, I will have to interact with other people, and they might not all be the friendliest people. So, I had to learn how to handle those types of situations in accordance with the word of God. He allowed me to go through some of the other situations that I did to increase my humility, empathy, compassion and ability to forgive.

I often wondered why I worked for long periods of time in such drastically different fields of employment. I worked in some form of customer service for over 20 years. But in addition to working in customer service I was a Bank Manager, a Billing Analyst, Accounting Representative, Project Manager, Billing Collection Officer, Housekeeper and Transcriptionist. Initially, I felt like I wasted a lot of valuable time in all of those different careers because I ended up having a career as a wellness coach, author and entrepreneur. I never saw any of those careers in my future and they are all vastly different from the careers and positions that I have held previously.

I felt the same way about the time and money that I invested in obtaining my Bachelor of Science in Management Degree and Project Management Certification, because I felt that I did not need to obtain that degree and certification to become an author and wellness coach. But one day God revealed that I will need all the experience that I acquired at each one of those jobs to manage my own company successfully in addition to the education and knowledge that I gained from obtaining my degree and certification because my life and my brand is the largest business and/or project that I can and will ever manage. God allowed me to remain in those positions to become proficient with various programs, work with diverse groups of individuals and master a wide array of skills so that I would be well prepared in every aspect to be successful when he blessed me with the opportunity. He allowed me to see the dangers of alcohol use and how low and far out of character it could take someone so that I would no longer use it as a coping mechanism and refer to Him and His word instead. He knew that allowing me to witness first-hand some less than favorable living quarters would spark the humanitarian in me to fight for and support change for better, safer, and cleaner living conditions for others. He was well aware that because of "my bleeding heart" for love, peace, equality, and acceptance that I would use my gift and voice to help and advocate for individuals like myself and loved ones who may live with mental health issues, learning disabilities, struggle with their weight, battle with alcohol or substance use disorder or be part of the LGBTQIA+ community.

Another lesson I learned was that I truly needed to become the change that I wished to see in the church and the world. I let some of those less than favorable experiences that I had at church cause me to feel bitter, become judgmental and unaccepting of people who thought and acted differently than I did. I even let some of those experiences and others make me question my religion (not my faith in God, solely my religion) and consider no longer going to church to worship because I could not believe that some Christians would treat others in that manner. But I learned that I do not know and understand everything nor do I need to. It was none of my business why some people behaved the way that they did. Like I have mentioned before, I have to constantly remind myself that I was attending church for Him (and His word, teaching and fellowship) not them. I needed to stay in alignment with the way God instructs us to respond to adversity in His word and not pass judgment.

Lastly, one of the most valuable lessons of all is that I learned self-control. In the end the only thing that I do have control over is how I respond in those challenging situations. I cannot let the actions of others dictate how I will react and respond. I have to remember that I am the daughter of a king and maintain a high level of dignity and respect for myself and others at all times. One of the best ways to promote change is to lead by example.

God has blessed me with the wisdom and favor to operate in my gift and purpose. Operating in my gift and purpose can and will propel me into my dream life. Listening and responding to His call, believing in His plan and following my strategy led me to create and develop my program, write my first book and create my brand. I gained the necessary skills, knowledge, and experience that I needed to execute my vision. I worked hard to build the foundation to sustain my brand and dream by changing and rebuilding my core. I now have to increase my faith to the maximum level to shatter through the glass ceiling to become the best version of me possible. I must truly understand and believe in the endless power of faith and the heights it can take me to when I listen, trust and obey His word to unlock his overflowing abundance of favor in my life. The time has come to create my vision board, pray, have faith and know that God will manifest my dreams.

As drastically as my life has changed over the years, so have my dreams. I was never a person who dreamed about being famous, being ridiculously rich or possessing an absurd amount of material things. My dreams were always about helping others, making a difference in my community and having peace and joy in my heart. The part of my dream about having joy and peace in my heart has remained the same but the focus and range has changed. I now dream about making a global impact in the world by helping people transform and improve their quality of life with a holistic approach through my books and coaching. Until recently, I never thought in my wildest dreams that I would ever write a book. Now looking back over my life, I can't believe I did not write a book sooner because several people over the years told me that I had the gift of writing including my family, elementary school teachers, professors and my pastor.

When they initially told me that writing was my gift, I thought they were just being kind and even if I did have the gift of writing, how could I use it to make a difference? I did not personally know any writers, so I was unsure how this "gift" would help or lead me to my purpose or dream. As I started to develop a stronger and more personal relationship with God, I started to hear more and more about "gifts" and the fact that God gave everyone a gift to fulfill their purpose and achieve their dreams. I knew that I could do a lot of different things on what I felt was a mediocre level, but nothing stood out to me as being my "gift" (even though I had been told point blank that my gift was writing, I still wasn't convinced).

One day I was watching some inspirational videos on YouTube and came across a speech by Steve Harvey titled Jump. In this video Steve Harvey said that if anyone is having trouble identifying their God given gift, they can identify their gift by determining what "thing" they do the absolute best with the least amount of effort.

He went on to say that when you find your gift it will lead you to operate in your purpose and help guide you to your passion to reach your dreams (or at least that is what I gathered from it). I immediately bought and read his book, also titled Jump where he further discussed this theory. During the time that I saw this video and read this book, I had been praying that God would clearly reveal and propel me into my purpose because I knew that the career that I was in was not my purpose.

I had begun to feel very anxious and unsettled at work. I had a very hard time concentrating and I could not stop thinking about what my purpose truly was. I felt like life was passing me by. This feeling reminded me of a quote by Les Brown, "The graveyard is the richest place on earth, because it is here that you will find all the hopes and dreams that were never fulfilled, the books that were never written, the songs that were never sung, the inventions that were never shared, the cures that were never discovered, all because someone was too afraid to take that first step, keep with the problem or determined to carry out their dream." I did not want to meet that fate and never fulfill my purpose or live my dream. So I am determined to do everything in my power to make sure that they come to fruition.

I had always been passionate about health and wellness, so I decided to start taking classes to earn my Holistic Wellness Coaching Certificate. Once I received my certification, I started working on developing my program and building my coaching business, but it was not an easy feat. I did not have a huge social media following because I rarely engaged in social media and had just moved to a new city from the small town that I grew up in a few years prior. Due to the pandemic I had been indoors and working from home for most of that timeframe. I had not had the opportunity to network and meet many new people so I had to come up with a plan B. I am confident that my program can truly help people and I needed to find a way to get it to the masses.

When I saw the Jump video by Steve Harvey and read his book by the same name that outlined how to identify your gift, I immediately knew that my gift was writing. In my previous roles as a Billing Analyst and Bank Manager, I have written entire training manuals for new hires and I wrote a weekly synopsis of the Sunday sermon for our church's website and social media platforms. I always receive compliments on what I have written and due to journaling daily writing has become second nature for me.

Instinctively, I decided to write a book about my holistic journey to wellness. I originally started writing the book with the plan that 70% of the book would cover intermittent fasting including what it is, how it works to heal the body, how it helps you to lose weight and sample meal plans made up of the foods that I consumed daily to lose over 70 pounds. About 10% of the book was going to be about my faith and how that guided me through my journey and in developing the program. The remaining 20% of the book was going to be about how I "shattered through the glass ceiling" overcame obstacles, broke through barriers, changed my core and increased my faith to increase God's favor. However, as I discussed earlier in the book God had a different plan. I always loved the saying "If you want to hear God laugh, tell him your plans."

After being diagnosed with Bipolar Affective Disorder and my experience in the days immediately following my diagnosis, my entire focus for the book shifted. I believe that God wanted me to write the book primarily about the obstacles that I overcame and how I did it by faith, praying and believing in Him and His word. When I had the vision of a hand erasing all of the letters I's out of my partially finished manuscript for the original book I was going to write and reflected on some of things that he brought back to the forefront of my mind that I had buried, I knew that He was leading me to tell my personal story to help others and not just write a book about the intermittent fasting and weight loss. He also wanted me to tell more about how He covered me and led me through the entire process. I must admit I was reluctant at first to share so much detail. I prayed for Him to confirm that I was receiving His message and instructions clearly and accurately.

Soon after that prayer, I started to receive more confirmation than I could handle from many different sources. Confirmation like people confiding in me that they had so much trauma and pain buried and it was starting to have a negative impact on their life and people telling me they needed someone to talk to who could relate to what they had been through or currently going through. I had two different people on separate occasions tell me that their mental health was in such bad shape that they had put getting a therapist or counselor on their Christmas list this year. This was all confirmation that there was a need for my book. In no way am I insinuating that my book or coaching sessions can replace the care of a licensed therapist or counselor but my book and services do help individuals identify their barriers and help them gain the confidence to face and overcome them. It lets them know that it is ok to not be ok and that they are not alone.

I received my assignment and confirmation from Him so it was time to get busy using my gift to do God's work. My initial dream was to help people lose weight and live a healthier lifestyle in an effort to prevent and better manage disease and illness such as diabetes and congestive heart failure. My current dream is to build a global brand that will assist people in becoming the best version of themselves possible through holistic wellness and make the world a better place in the process. I know that achieving my dream requires radical faith and that is exactly what I have! (Matthew 7:7 "Ask and it will be given to you, seek and you will find, knock and the door will be opened to you." (Psalm 20:4 "May He give you the desire of your heart and make all your plans succeed").

Creating a plan and vision board list is the next step in Phase IV after identifying my gift, purpose and dream. Although having radical faith and God's will and favor will be huge components in achieving my dream, I have to work in alignment with Him and operate in a manner that coincides with my trust in His word that He will do what He says he will do because faith without works is dead (James 2:26 "As the body without the spirit is dead so faith without deeds is dead"). I will not write an enormous amount of detail on my vision board list because I understand and respect that God is in control and I do not have all of the answers, but it will be a visual reminder of my goals and plans to ensure that I stay focused and on track. I will approach my planning and vision board list from a holistic perspective also; Mind, Body and Spirit.

Writing this book was very therapeutic for me. I was able to do what is sometimes referred to as a "brain dump" in the therapy world and spring clean my mind, clearing out all of the clutter. It allowed me to share my journey with others who may be facing some of the same challenges, obstacles and barriers that I did and offer help and hope that we can take our power back, heal and change our circumstances. I believe that this book has the potential to truly change anyone's life who reads it. Because of that reason, I plan to heavily promote this book. I invested in my dream and published independently so that I could maintain creative control and ensure that my vision for the book and brand came to life just the way that I imagined and God instructed. I pray that I am invited to speak all over the country on mega platforms such as TBN, Oprah's Soulful Sundays, Tamron Hall, The Tyler Perry Show and everywhere else possible to get the message in this book out in the world. I will continue my book tour and do as many speaking engagements as God leads and allows me to do.

I intend to write several more books in the Elegant Elevation Self Help Book series to provide more issue specific information and help on topics that my readers struggle with. Self-help books for the youth and young adults that will be under the Elegant Elevation umbrella but will be categorized as titles for Generation Z are next on my agenda. These books will explain how to deal with the daily challenges that our youth face from a biblical perspective. Since it seems like God has been taken out of our schools, communities and work environments, I want to do my part to invite Him back in. Getting my feet wet in the fiction writing pool is also on my to-do list.

I also plan to have a coordinating apparel and novelty items line that offers articles such as shirts, purses, masks, hats, coffee mugs, coasters and pens that reference some of my favorite Bible scriptures that were mentioned in this book. The coordinating items would reference scriptures on them such as Matthew 25:40, but the apparel will have M.25:40 or 25:40 on it. I think this is a creative way to promote reading the Bible and absorbing His word again. Who wants to have or carry an item and they do not know what it is saying or referencing. I know if I saw scripture that I did not recognize or know by heart on an item, out of curiosity I would definitely go immediately look it up so that I would understand the meaning and why that person was promoting that specific scripture. I would know that it must have some significant meaning in that person's life. I also plan to expand my online coaching services and have various resources available at the fingertips of people who need it.

Since our body is a temple, I wholeheartedly believe that we should care for it as such. I shared my plan to practice better self-care in the Phase III section of this book, but I also want to continue to help and coach others to do the same on a broader scale. I want to make sure that the clients that I coach know that they do not have to step foot in a gym in order to live a healthy lifestyle and lose weight. I lost over 70 pounds and never had a gym membership. The important part of exercise is that you are moving your body continuously for at least thirty consecutive minutes five times a week and that you do something that you enjoy doing so you look forward to exercising (not dread it) and stay consistent. I lost all of my weight by power walking outside in my neighborhood while listening to music and podcasts, doing my old Shaun T Hip Hop Abs and Rockin' Body DVDs and following a Walk at Home program by Leslie Sansone (The Walk at Home app is about $5.00 month and offers hundreds of workouts). There is absolutely nothing wrong with going to the gym or hiring a trainer. However, I just want to provide my clients with options if they are not comfortable going to the gym, don't have the time or extra money to afford a gym membership or a personal trainer. We do not have to follow what everyone else is doing or the latest trend to lose weight and get healthy. We can do that in the privacy of our own homes if we choose to.

Once my book launches and a "few" more people know who I am I will pitch my idea to create an Elegant Elevation (EE) fitness tracker or an EE version of an existing high quality tracker. I absolutely love my Fitbit and all of the useful data that it tracks, such as my sleep habits, heart rate, steps and miles walked each day, water intake and menstrual cycle. However, I believe that some of the data collected should populate in currency (or have the ability to be converted to currency) instead of numbers to reflect the investment that you are making into your health when you practice healthy habits such as exercising, drinking water and getting adequate sleep. I believe it is a fun and creative way to show the value of investing in your health and wellness to become the best version of you. Many people would get a thrill from seeing the dollar amount increase throughout the day versus seeing a step count. Even though technically it would not be "real money" it would encourage people to be more active and practice healthy habits just to see their currency increase. (Just think about the last game of monopoly that you played with your family). Health is our greatest wealth and tools like fitness trackers should illustrate that.

I also plan to pitch a TV show idea that would be a mix between The Biggest Loser, Dancing with the Stars, My 600-Pound Life and Iyanla Fix My Life. The core concept of the show would be the same as my book Elegant Elevation which is helping people become the best versions of themselves. The contestants/clients would compete in a competition to lose the highest percentage of their body weight. But they would also get the opportunity to deal with any underlying issues that caused them to overeat or gain weight in the first place by using faith and the word of God as weapons of warfare to shatter through the glass ceiling and overcome their obstacles and challenges. There would be licensed therapists and/ or counselors available for the contestants/clients to talk with and assist them with breaking through any barriers that have prevented them from losing weight and maintaining weight loss in the past. There would be four coaches on the show. My dream cast would be myself, Shaun T, Tabitha Brown and Kenya Crooks. I selected this specific cast for four main reasons: (1) Each one of us is a believer in God. (2) Each one of us is passionate about health and wellness. (3) Each one of us has a unique and bold personality. (4) Each one of us promotes a different eating style and approach to wellness.

All of these components make for good television. Shaun T is also an open and proud member of the LGBTQIA+ community. As discussed previously in this book, I would love to help remove the stigma around being a part of the LGBTQIA+community and being a believer. My hope would be that a show like that would take the focus off our differences and focus on a common enemy which is obesity and it doesn't discriminate.

Diseases and illnesses directly related to obesity are killing people in every demographic at an alarming rate, so regardless of who loses the highest percentage of body weight on the show, everyone's a winner because we are all working together towards a common goal to fight and win the war against obesity. Each coach would have a male and a female contestant to work with who would follow their coach's eating plan and exercise regime. There would be a weigh in each week to gauge the progress of each team. At home viewers would be able to participate by following the plan of their choice or their favorite coach and use social media to vote for their favorite team.

After each weigh in the contestants would have the choice to either stay with their original team and coach or switch to another team. Before every weigh in everyone would participate in the weekly "round table" session where the contestants would write down the issues and obstacles they dealt with for that week and we would all discuss as an entire group with the coaches weighing in and giving advice. The contestants can be as vague or as detailed as they would like as they describe their issues in an effort to protect their privacy. At the conclusion of the "round table" session we would throw the papers that they wrote the obstacles on into the "prayer pit" and pray together over each of those issues as a group (Matthew 18:19 "Again, truly I tell you that if two of you on earth agree about anything they ask for, it will be done for them by my Father in heaven").

Some may wonder why I am writing and sharing my vision and ideas. The reason is because I wanted to be completely transparent and share my entire journey to becoming the best version of me, so that others can have a clear understanding and can apply the steps in this program to do the same. I have been asked if I was afraid someone would "steal my ideas". My answer is no. God put these ideas in my heart and although I am passionate about personally fulfilling them, if someone else is able to take them and use them, then it just means it wasn't meant for me to do it. What He has for me is for me and no one will be able to take that. And if someone else does make a show like this come to fruition I am still a winner because it could and would help so many people. This is a huge dream of mine because obesity has robbed so many of us of our loved ones. It would be a unique and enjoyable way to address the obesity epidemic as a collective effort, united front and use the television platform to increase awareness. We spend so much time debating about our differences that we neglect to put the necessary effort into collaborating to fight our common enemies, like obesity, mental and behavioral health issues, unfair treatment of those who live with disabilities and God being removed from our schools, work environments, and sadly enough even from some of our churches. It would be beautiful to work together as believers to fight a common enemy.

The spirit component is the most important component as it relates to increasing our faith to become the best version of ourselves. I mentioned earlier in this book that I planned on becoming a more active member in my church and sharing my gifts and talents as much as possible. I plan to suggest and/or spearhead forming a couples/ready to marry/marriage ministry at our church. When our pastor conducted a series on marriage last year it was extremely popular and the congregation was extremely interactive. The response to that series demonstrated that there was an interest and need for that ministry in our church. We are currently a small church but most of the members are married. I believe that we could all benefit from sharing our experiences of what has worked and what has not in our marriage, how we have overcome barriers and obstacles and the overall fellowship. I did not want the "marriage ministry" to be exclusive because there are some singles that are looking to get married and some couples who may be engaged that could learn and benefit from engaging in fellowship with married couples. We also have a wide age range of members in our congregation that are in different stages of their marriage such as recently married, married for 20+ years and some couples have been married for over 50 years. I believe that each couple would have some valuable information and knowledge to share with others members of the congregation. I would like to see this ministry meet once a month or every other month and rotate between having game nights, open discussion, group date nights, and visit and participate in other churches' marriage ministry events in the community.

Another goal as it relates to the spirit component is to have this book become a resource for my home church and other churches to counsel their members on various issues that have been historically either avoided or proven challenging for the church to address. I would love for this book to be used as part of the new members' class curriculum. I believe that this book could help new members shatter through barriers and overcome obstacles early on so that they would be more confident as a believer and a stronger soldier in God's army.

I plan to give back to both pastors who helped me tremendously grow in my faith and mature as a Christian woman. My former pastor always spoke of his plans to one day build a youth resource and recreational center on the same lot that the church currently resides on. He wanted to provide the youth with a safe place to come, be productive and socialize with other believers. He wanted to offer tutoring, mentoring and sports for the kids to participate in, with the hope that having a positive outlet would prevent them from getting into trouble. Most of the youth in our small community have a tremendous amount of talent and the potential to be great. As the crimes committed by and to the youth in the small town continue to rise at an accelerated pace, these programs and resources are desperately needed. I plan to give a donation to that effort as soon as I am financially able to.

My current pastor is an amazing visionary, teacher and leader. He has taught me so much over the last few years about the Bible and having the ability to understand various Greek and Hebrew translations. I have to admit, I used to at times avoid going to Sunday school and Bible study because it could be challenging to follow along and get a clear understanding of the scriptures and the material that was being presented. My pastor has shown me how to decipher the material so that I can fully comprehend the information and now I truly enjoy attending those classes. Our church is located in a great up and coming neighborhood, but the church is in need of a slight facelift and a few minor updates and repairs. I also plan to make a significant donation towards those renovations.

I have completed the four phases of my Elegant Elevation program to become the best version of me through faith, fasting and God's favor. I have shared a detailed depiction of how I transformed my mess into a message, my trials in triumphs and my tests into a testimony. I am confident that with God's help and guidance you can and will do the same to become the best version of you. The only deeds left to do after completing the four phases of my Elegant Elevation program are to keep working in alignment with His will, increase my trust and faith in Him and continue to praise Him for what He has already done and what He is going to do in my life.

CONCLUSION

The first step in the Elegant Elevation program is determining why you want and need to become the best version of you. My reason for wanting to become the best version of me was knowing that God called me to be greater. My loved ones and the people I want to help deserve that version of me. Everyone's journey to holistic wellness and becoming the best version of themselves is going to be unique. Our backgrounds, barriers, obstacles, gifts and goals are all different. However, the necessary components of faith, intermittent fasting and God's favor are universal. Even if your goal is not to lose weight, fasting can be a helpful tool in providing clarity in your life. Some of us can also benefit from fasting from other vices besides food to allow more time to hear from God and allow the Holy Spirit to move in our lives.

The phases of the Elegant Elevation program will be the same for everyone despite our individual goals and barriers. In order for us to shatter through the glass ceiling to become the best version of ourselves we need to complete all four phases of the program. This book provides a step by step guide through each phase of my journey to shattering through my glass ceiling to become the best version of me. I started by determining what past and present obstacles have hindered me from becoming the best version of me.

We must identify the source of our pain and our barriers in order to overcome them (Phase I: Stop the Bleeding/Find the Source). In this phase I identified and made a list of the major barriers that hindered me from becoming the best version of me. The next phase is to overcome our barriers and heal from the pain that those barriers caused (Phase II: Remove the Debris/Purify Your Heart). In this phase I acknowledged and confessed those barriers. I opened my heart and prayed for God's forgiveness, grace, mercy and favor to help me shatter through those barriers and to grant me a clean heart. The third phase is leaving the pain behind and becoming a new you (Phase III: Change and Rebuild Your Core). During this phase I began to design the person I wanted to become by changing my way of thinking and heart in addition to developing a healthier and more holistic approach to wellness including mind, body and spirit. The final phase of the Elegant Elevation Program is becoming stronger and more confident in your faith to manifest your dream life (Phase IV: Strengthen Your Faith to Become the Best Version of You). In the final phase I began to truly believe in myself and trust the power of God. I started to chase my dreams and live more fearlessly, knowing that with God in my life, all things are possible.

The Elegant Elevation transformation process is not a destination. It is a journey and hopefully you will always want to continue to grow and evolve into the best version of you. May God keep you and bless your life abundantly!

ACKNOWLEDGEMENTS

To my husband, thank you for being my rock through this entire process and consistently cheering me on during this rollercoaster ride we call life, love, and marriage. I know that it isn't always easy. I love and cherish you babe.

To my oldest daughter, thank you for your patience and understanding while I tried to figure this thing called motherhood out. I am so proud of you and the mother and advocate for others that you have become. I love you to the moon and back.

To my youngest daughter, thank you for always being there to listen and hold my hand. I am so proud of the beautiful soul that you are and how dedicated you are to helping the intellectually challenged and disabled community. I love you through the stars and beyond.

To my only son, thank you for being unapologetically you. You never let my fears hold you back from living life to the fullest and on your terms and you encourage others to do the same. I love you more than words could ever express.

To my gbabies thank you for giving me another opportunity to enjoy the amazing and fun parts of motherhood. I love you all with my entire heart and soul.

To my older sister, thank you for being a trailblazer for the family and working to break generational curses to bring our family closer together. I love you big sis.

To my younger sister, thank you for sometimes acting like the older sister and having those difficult conversations with me that I did not want to hear or have at the time but needed to. I love you baby girl.

To all of my family, friends, pastors, fellow church members and co-workers who poured and sowed into me over the years and saw in me what I couldn't and didn't see in myself. Thank you from the bottom of my heart. I love you.

<u>**For Interviews, Speaking Engagements or Coaching Services,**</u>
<u>**Please Contact Me At:**</u>

<u>septembermichelle@yahoo.com</u>

Facebook: Michelle R. Williams

Instagram: @elegant_elevation07_

Twitter: @ElegntElevation

Printed in the United States
by Baker & Taylor Publisher Services